THE HEALTHY WOMAN

Helen Buckler
Dept of
Endocrinology
Hope
Hospital

Dedicated to
the late Jean Hailes and the women of Australia

The Healthy Woman

Better health management and the menopause

Susan Davis MBBS, FRACP, PhD

with contributions from
Professor Henry Burger, Dr Elizabeth Farrell, Professor David Healy,
Ms Assunta Hunter, Dr Diane Palmer

FOR THE JEAN HAILES FOUNDATION

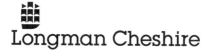

Longman Cheshire

DISCLAIMER

The information contained in this book is intended to be a guide for women. Neither Dr Susan Davis nor the publisher can accept responsibility for your health or any side-effects of the treatments outlined in this book. You should always be guided by your own doctor when following any treatment whether it be conventional or natural therapy.

Thanks to Jenny Coopes
for the cartoons.

Longman Cheshire Pty Limited
Longman House
Kings Gardens
95 Coventry Street
Melbourne 3205 Australia

Offices in Sydney, Brisbane, Adelaide and Perth, and associated companies throughout the world.

Designed by Rob Cowpe
Cover designed by Rob Cowpe
Produced by Longman Cheshire Pty Ltd
Set in 11/13pt Adobe Garamond
Printed in Australia

National Library of Australia
Cataloguing-in-Publication data

Davis, Susan (Susan Ruth), 1957-
    The healthy woman: better health management and the Menopause

    ISBN 0 582 80226 1.
    1. Menopause—Popular works. I. Jean Hailes Menopause Foundation. II. Title

618.175

FOREWORD

It is more than twelve years since Jean Hailes published her monograph on the menopause. Since then much has been written—the menopause is now recognised as an event in women's lives that is freely discussed by women (and men) as a change that may be expected as part of middle age.

In this monograph, Dr Susan Davis, mother of four young children (and by no means middle-aged), has taken over from Jean Hailes who died in 1979. Dr Davis has expanded on many aspects of the menopause and has taken advantage of discoveries made over the past ten to fifteen years.

She has also enlisted the aid of other health professionals with certain sections of the book. One of these, a completely new section, describes the use of natural therapies and provides some warning about placing too much reliance on such treatments.

In taking over from Jean Hailes, Susan Davis has filled the need to provide simple, clear explanations and advice about how best to deal with what may for some be a difficult period. She recognises the need for counselling, even for those women who experience few, if any, difficulties at that time. She provides reassurance for such women for whom hormone replacement therapy is neither necessary nor indicated.

Dr Bryan Hudson
Founding Professor of Medicine, Monash University
and former Director of the Howard Florey Institute for Experimental Physiology & Medicine

PREFACE

I was originally asked by the publisher to revise Jean Hailes' book *The Middle Years,* first published in 1980. Jean's book was clear, concise and informative and written for women in their middle years by someone who cared very much for other women. I could never presuppose that I could reproduce Jean's light humorous style, she wrote as she spoke. That would be presumptuous. Therefore with the encouragement of Jean Hailes' family, particularly her daughter, Janet Hailes Michelmore, I have put together this manuscript which provides fundamental health information for Australian women.

This manuscript has been prepared with the invaluable assistance of several other people. I would like to thank Dr Diane Palmer, Professor Henry Burger, Professor David Healy, Dr Elizabeth Farrell, Ms Assunta Hunter and Dr Robyn Craven.

I am also indebted to Dr Bryan Hudson, formerly Foundation Professor of Medicine, Monash University and past Director of The Howard Florey Institute, who has been my mentor for many years.

Susan Davis
DECEMBER 1993

CONTENTS

INTRODUCTION

This book was written with the philosophy that the menopause is a natural event in every woman's life. The pre-menopausal and the post-menopausal years reflect gradual changes that occur in a woman's body as a result of the menopause. These changes are natural but are modified by each woman's characteristics and the interaction with her environment. Each woman is a unique biological entity and just as puberty is experienced in varying ways by different women so is the menopause. About ten per cent of women are significantly disabled by this change in their hormones but for the majority it is a minor inconvenience. Thus we must not dismiss the severe symptoms some women experience, nor should we label all midlife women as diseased!

As a result of improved nutrition, hygiene and medical intervention the life expectancy of Western women is approximately eighty years. Since most women can expect to live at least one third of their lives after their menopause it is vital to have the best possible physical and mental health in order to have maximum quality of life in these years. There is a clearly desirable broad spectrum of attitudes towards the menopause within the general public, the scientific community, the medical fraternity and allied health providers. Some even take opposing 'sides' and attempt to categorise people into those who see menopause as a hormone deficiency disease that must be treated medically and those who view it as a natural transition which requires no intervention. Such perspectives are not only extreme but also unhelpful. It is an irrefutable fact that menopause results in a reduction in the production of hormones from the ovaries, and relative to the reproductive years post-menopausal women are deficient in these hormones.

The concept that menopause is a normal biological event does not exclude the use of medical or alternative therapy. Fertility for women is normal and yet these days contraception in its many forms is acceptable. Medical intervention is used in many ways to make life more comfortable as well as to treat distinct diseases, and so it is an option for the post-menopausal woman.

So the basis for this book is to give women a background from which to make their own choice.

My aim is to provide women with information about their own biology, the menopause in general, and the short- and long-term consequences of the menopause. Armed with information, each woman will be able to seek out and consider the options available to her and make her own choices. *The needs and choices of the individual are paramount and preventative measures, natural therapies and hormone replacement are not mutually exclusive.* The options are numerous and each woman must take into account her own immediate needs, for example symptoms, future health prospects, including risks of osteoporosis or cardiovascular disease, and lifestyle expectations, when considering the appropriateness of hormone replacement therapy.

Extremist propaganda should be viewed with a moderate degree of cynicism. Statements such as 'All menopausal women should take hormone replacement therapy' and 'Hormone replacement therapy is a male medical and pharmaceutical manipulation of middle-aged women', are equally ridiculous, as well as frightening. It is more realistic to have a balanced approach and an open mind when dealing with personal issues whether they relate to health or relationships. When it comes to making decisions about dealing with menopause and related problems, seek out information and help. Discuss the issues that are important to you and be active in making decisions regarding your therapy.

I believe the aim of every woman transiting the menopause should be to have optimal health and well-being so as to enjoy her middle years and beyond. I hope the information that follows will enable women to choose for themselves how best to handle this transition.

Chapter 1

THE EXPERIENCE OF THE MENOPAUSE TRANSITION

The menopause is a normal biological event in every woman's life when the ovaries no longer produce eggs and hormones. However, there is enormous variation in how women experience and view the transition both in physical terms and in terms of its effect on their psyche or social life. Menopause is perceived and experienced very differently by individuals in the same community and by those who live in different cultures in general. Health and a woman's attitude towards health are influenced by the immediate environment and the culture within which she operates. Culture will alter the experience of menopause because of the effect it has on determining a woman's lifestyle and expectations—diet, whether or not it is acceptable to smoke or drink alcohol, how many children a woman has and so on, are all influenced by her culture. The interpretation of the significance of menstruation and fertility varies greatly between populations and reflects directly on how a particular society interprets the menopause.

There are some factors in an individual woman's biological make-up which may determine the experience she will have at the time of the menopause. After menopause the ovary is no longer the major source of oestrogen and the amount of oestrogen produced in other parts of the body, particularly in fat tissue, varies greatly between women. Different levels in oestrogen between post–menopausal women may partially account for the variations in symptoms experienced by women during the menopausal transition. Women with more fat tissue generally have higher oestrogen levels and so there may be some value in a controlled 'middle-aged spread'.

While these biological factors may be very important they are only the beginning of multiple and interconnecting factors that work together to account for the menopause experience for an individual woman. Other than the cessation of periods, which happens to all women as the ovary no longer produces hormones, the most common symptom reported by women is the hot flush. In Western developed countries like Australia, hot flushes are reported by about seventy per cent of women but only about ten per cent will describe them as severe. The women who seek medical help for their hot flushes are not necessarily those with the worst symptoms. It has been shown in research in Australia and overseas, it is more likely that *hot flushes in association with psychological stress will influence a woman to seek medical help.*

In other countries the rate of reporting of hot flushes is different. For example, in some Asian countries symptoms are reported less frequently than in Western countries. In Japan there is no word in the language which corresponds to the meaning of hot flush—in one study Japanese women were most likely to report stiff shoulders as the most common symptom they related to menopause. Similarly, traditional Malaysian and Hong Kong women are unlikely to seek medical treatment for the menopause. Several studies including women in Hong Kong, Karachi and Indonesia reveal that *anxiety about menopause symptoms is more likely to occur with increasing affluence and exposure to Western culture.* There is no simple explanation as to why Asian women experience the menopause differently. Contributing factors probably include the general attitude of their society towards older women and lifestyle, especially differences between the Western and traditional Asian diet.

The effect of cultural background

A woman's culture will usually influence family size and a woman's life can vary across cultures from one of many pregnancies followed by long periods of breast-feeding, to one of many regular menstrual cycles interrupted only by the occasional pregnancy. This variability does not seem to have any effect on the *age* of menopause—this has remained remarkably constant across cultures and through the centuries at about fifty. How this variation affects the *experience* of the menopause has not been adequately assessed but there has been no obvious pattern identified to date.

The expected life span of a woman varies dramatically between countries and is clearly related to differing health and living standards. The symptoms of the menopause, or any long-term consequences, may have little importance if the life expectancy of a woman is not much more than the average age of menopause.

The heightened awareness of the menopause in more affluent Western societies may partly result from high health expectations and increased life expectancy.

In Australia in the 1990s the average life expectancy for women is about eighty years so that a large proportion of women will live almost a third of their lives after the menopause. For Koori women, however, the picture is unfortunately very different—in 1988 the life expectancy for Koori women in rural New South Wales was only fifty-two years. For these women health issues are related to the problems of heart disease, diabetes and respiratory diseases and the menopause has little relevance.

In Pakistan the life expectancy of a woman is now fifty-eight years but as recently as twenty-five years ago the average Pakistani woman was only expected to live to the age of forty-four. Clearly many women were never fortunate enough to reach the age of menopause and neither the symptoms nor the long-term consequences of menopause were significant in comparison to other health issues in Pakistan's society. Now, as women in Pakistan and other underdeveloped countries are living longer, the menopause and its long-term effects are now being considered as major issues with respect to women's health.

The culture in which a woman lives will also determine her lifestyle to a large extent. In less developed cultures a woman's life is likely to involve much more physical activity. Research has demonstrated that regular exercise will be associated with improvements in health including the reduction of frequency of hot flushes and risk of development of osteoporosis and cardiovascular disease. Certain cultures will traditionally have a diet that contains more plant oestrogens which may decrease the frequency of hot flushes as will the use of traditional Chinese herbal medicines which can contain oestrogen-like substances.

Perhaps, however, the most important influence a culture has on a woman's experience of the menopause is in the way the culture views women and the importance of their fertility, and its attitude in general to ageing. In Asian cultures the menopause is regarded as a natural event and women are not apprehensive of its onset. There is no sense of foreboding for the coming of old age because people of advanced age are highly respected and considered competent and dignified. The loss of fertility is welcomed as the removal of the continuous threat of further pregnancies, and the menopause is seen as almost graduating (up?) to male status! In societies where menstrual blood is feared as a contaminant, there are many taboos and restrictions that are applied to menstruating women and release from these taboos can be extremely liberating both socially and emotionally. Occasionally, in some cultures, this time of life can bring an almost mystical status as post-menopausal women are thought to possess healing and supernatural powers. Alternatively, in a youth-orientated society, it may be seen only in terms of losses.

A study of Mayan women in Mexico found that these women had a lifestyle involving much physical exercise, a diet low in fat and protein, many pregnancies and in middle age they gained importance as the heads of their married sons' extended households. These women had a very positive attitude to menopause and old age—welcoming it and feeling free to enjoy the tranquillity associated with it—they report no symptoms of the menopause other than cessation of periods. In India the Rajput women of Rajistan are freed from the custom of wearing the veil of Purdah at the menopause and are seen as equal to men and no longer able to contaminate with their menstrual blood. They report few symptoms at the menopause. In contrast the Mashona women of south east Zimbabwe experience a dramatic loss of status at the menopause. Being no longer able to bear children they may be discarded by their husbands who want fertile younger wives and may face a very precarious situation dependent on the benevolence of their children. Mashona women have a high rate of reporting symptoms at the menopause.

Most Western societies studied also have a relatively high reporting rate of symptoms although the majority of women in community studies do not regard their troublesome symptoms as abnormal. Several studies have suggested that menopause is 'no big deal' from an overall community perspective, as opposed to what is apparent from studies of women attending menopause clinics.

Amid hopes that it will change, Western society has been cruelly youth-orientated and sexist. The middle-aged woman has often been a figure of ridicule (no one likes being called an 'old woman') and is often ignored completely. Middle-aged women can feel they are invisible as the world around them fails to acknowledge them simply because they are no longer seen as (sexually) attractive. It is no wonder that there is a pervasive fear of ageing amongst women.

Our Western society has developed a tragic caricature of the older woman. She is depicted as inept, rigid in her outlook, with undesirable physical changes such as:

- grey hair
- wrinkles
- drooping breasts
- balding
- facial hair
- fat or thin but never in-between, and
- finally seen as being asexual

Some women will do anything to avoid such physical changes whereas others sadly resign themselves to the 'ageing' process and almost give up trying to look their best. It has been suggested also that loss of social status may well be related to an increased rate of symptom reporting at the menopause.

There has been some concern expressed by workers in Asian countries that increasing Westernisation may increase the reporting rate of symptoms although as yet there is no clear pattern emerging to support this fear. Care must be taken not to generalise so that the menopause is defined as a medical syndrome created by Western society. Only recently is its significance to women from different cultures being studied and understood.

Effects of social and personal background

While the negative cultural stereotype of menopause and middle age will impact on most women's lives within a culture the effect it has on the experience of an individual woman will also depend on other factors. It has been shown in American and British studies that women are more likely to find the menopause associated with troublesome symptoms if they have a low socio-economic status, a low education level or are unemployed. An Australian study being conducted in Melbourne has found a higher symptom reporting rate in women who have chronic health problems, in those who had premenstrual or menstrual complaints in the past and in those who have interpersonal stress problems and less positive attitudes to menopause and ageing.

> The interactions of stress and menopausal symptoms are very complex.

It was found in a Sydney study that there was no difference in the reported rate of troublesome symptoms between women who sought medical help and those that did not—however what was different between the groups was that the women seeking help had a higher rate of stress-related problems. Similar studies overseas have suggested that lower self-esteem is characteristic of women who seek medical help at the menopause. Mid-life can be a time of great stress. Coping with problems with adolescents, with death of parents, non-attainment of career goals or, more frequently in recent years, retrenchment and unemployment. There is some research to suggest that changes in hormone levels may have direct effects on brain function and mood. Given the complexity of the interrelationships that can develop it is difficult to isolate effects of the menopause alone. It may be that hormonal changes at the menopause make women more vulnerable to stress factors and that women who are already stressed find the addition of troublesome symptoms hard to bear. Women whose menopause occurs prematurely (before forty years of age), are one group who may have particular problems especially if this occurs before they are able to have the children they would love to have.

> It is important that emphasis be given to the fact that *for the majority of women mid-life is not a negative experience,* that despite the presence of symptoms *menopausal women in the main regard themselves as healthy.* Some will feel better than they have in their whole life and may discover the post-menopausal zest that anthropologist Margaret Mead described as 'the most creative force in the world'.

Chapter 2

THE MENOPAUSE— WHAT DOES IT MEAN?

The menopause is a 'normal life event' and should be seen as a time of transition from the reproductive years into the productive years of adult life. It is a phase when a woman can reap the benefits of her formative years and enjoy what she has already established. Alternatively it can be a time for a fresh start—an opportunity to do things she has always hoped to do but been unable to because of constraints such as family responsibilities. For many women in careers it coincides with the opportunity to maximise their career potential. Just as puberty introduces women into a new and exciting phase of life, menopause should be viewed as another time of change and a gateway to a positive future.

Unfortunately, however, in general Australian society the word 'menopause' signifies the end of a woman's reproductive life and in our Western culture this has an overwhelmingly negative connotation. The formal medical definition of the menopause determined by the World Health Organisation is 'The permanent cessation of menstruation, resulting from the loss of ovarian follicular activity'. This means that the ovaries have completed their reproductive function and no longer produce mature eggs for ovulation each month. In simpler terms '*The menopause' is the last menstrual period.* In Caucasian women over the age of forty-five, it can be assumed with ninety per cent certainty that the menopause is established after twelve months without menstruation.

Most women have their last period between the ages of forty-five and fifty-five. Only five per cent continue to menstruate after fifty-three years of age.

What Happens to 'The Hormones'?

A baby girl is born with approximately six to seven million eggs. Menopause occurs when the ovaries run out of eggs. The majority of eggs deteriorate within the ovaries and never mature for ovulation, this is quite normal. The ovaries produce the hormones oestrogen (the major oestrogen being oestradiol) and progesterone each month during the process of egg maturation and ovulation. When there are no eggs left in the ovaries and ovulation ceases, so does the production of these hormones.

The ovaries also produce androgens which are more commonly known as the 'male hormones'. Androgens are believed to have an important biological role in women as well as in men. The major active androgen produced by the ovary is testosterone. During the normal menstrual cycle the level of testosterone in the blood increases at the time of ovulation. Following natural menopause the ovaries produce less testosterone. Some symptoms such as fatigue and lessened libido have been attributed to low post-menopausal androgen levels.

In the years or months leading to the menopause, hormone production by the ovaries may wax and wane. As a result *it is common for women to experience symptoms even though they are still menstruating.* Similarly the menstrual pattern often changes and cycles may become erratic, that is longer or shorter, and periods may be lighter or heavier. Most commonly the cycle length shortens in the years leading up to the menopause. This is due to the shortening of the first part of the cycle when an egg is developing for ovulation. Over the age of forty up to fifteen per cent of menstrual cycles do not result in the production of a mature egg. When menstrual irregularity develops in the pre-menstrual years a variety of hormonal patterns are observed, and there is no value in measuring hormonal levels at this stage. Some women may stop menstruating suddenly, without any prior irregularities in their cycles.

Why do periods stop?

The most identifiable menopausal experience for a woman is when menstruation ceases. Oestradiol stimulates the lining of the uterus to grow each month, ready for the possibility of conception. Progesterone modifies the uterine lining so it changes to a mature form in preparation for implantation of an embryo. If conception does not occur, the hormone levels suddenly fall and the lining is sloughed off in preparation for the next cycle. This is experienced as the monthly menstrual bleed. When the ovaries stop making oestradiol and progesterone the monthly changes in the uterus no longer occur and so periods cease.

Women who smoke cigarettes go through menopause on average eighteen months earlier than non-smokers. This is because nicotine has a toxic effect on the cells of the ovaries. Nicotine also affects the way in which the body metabolises oestrogen, and in general smokers have lower oestrogen levels throughout their reproductive life. Women who smoke are also likely to have lower than expected bone density (see chapter 3). This is the result of the nicotine having a toxic effect on bone cells, combined with smokers having lower oestrogen levels and earlier menopause.

Fertility and contraceptive options for the older woman

It is well known that a woman's fertility declines with increasing age. This decline becomes more marked after thirty-five and falls more rapidly after forty, when her potential fertility is fifty per cent of that at age twenty-five. This is due to a reduction in the number and quality of eggs produced by the ovary and to a decreasing ability of the ovary to respond to biochemical messages from the brain. It is also related to the reduced frequency of intercourse in older couples (with many exceptions). The menopause means the end of a woman's reproductive capacity but it is a diagnosis which cannot be made until twelve months after the last period. Any menstrual cycle up to and including the last one can be potentially fertile, however, and so pregnancy remains a lower but real risk. Pregnancy for women over forty carries increased risks to the mother's health and to the unborn baby. Complications of, for example, high blood pressure, pre-eclampsia (toxaemia) and pregnancy-related diabetes are more common in older women and this is so even in women who have no health problems prior to such a pregnancy. Miscarriage, foetal abnormality and still-birth are also more common but forty-five per cent of pregnancies will have a successful outcome.

An unplanned pregnancy is a very distressing event at any age but in an older woman it may be particularly stressful as it can be very unexpected, associated with the above risks and abortion may be less acceptable as an option to a woman who has had children. There is a generally lower use of contraception in this age group and a significant percentage of abortions is still performed in women over the age of thirty-five.

A general recommendation regarding contraception is that it be continued for a year after the last menstrual period if this occurs when a woman is over fifty, or for two years if she is less than fifty.

Menopausal symptoms may develop while a woman is still having menstrual cycles—some of which may be fertile. It must be remembered that Hormone Replacement Therapy as it is usually prescribed is not the same as the oral contraceptive pill and has not been demonstrated to be effective as a contraceptive.

The contraceptive choices available to an older woman are limited by factors in her medical history or lifestyle and not by any age-related problems of contraceptive methods. It used to be said that women over the age of thirty-five should not use the pill due to an increased risk of heart disease in older pill users. It has however been demonstrated that this increased risk is confined to women who smoke or who are in some other way at increased risk. *A woman who is well, does not smoke and who has no other risk factors for heart disease is now thought to be able to take the pill until the age of the menopause without any increased risk to her health.* The pill contains oestrogen which will also provide relief from hot flushes, maintain vaginal skin thickness and lubrication and conserve bone density.

Sterilisation remains the most popular method of contraception in this age group. The progesterone-only pill (minipill) and barrier methods (diaphragm/condom) also provide very effective contraception alternatives. It has been demonstrated that, consistent with lower fertility rates, the failure rate of any method of contraception is less than in younger women. 'Natural family planning' based on detection of cervical mucus changes and cycle predicability may be more difficult due to the increasing frequency of cycle irregularity.

Contraception for women at any age remains an issue about which she herself should make the final decision once she has access to information about effectiveness, benefits and side-effects of the various available methods.

Surgical menopause

If a woman has had her ovaries removed surgically then she is rendered immediately menopausal irrespective of her age. One of the earliest records of this surgery is from 1775 when Percival Pott described in the medical journal *Chirurgical Observations,* the menopausal changes experienced by a twenty-three year old woman whose ovaries were surgically removed—'she has enjoyed good health ever since, but has become thinner and apparently more muscular, her breasts which were large are gone; nor has she menstruated since the operation, which is now some years'. The most common medical reason for such an operation in a pre-menopause woman is endometriosis.

A woman who has had a hysterectomy only and the ovaries are not removed will continue to have normal function of the ovaries and oestradiol and progesterone are produced in the normal way. However, *menopause does occur earlier in women who have had a hysterectomy.* One of the theories for this is that the blood supply to the ovaries may have been disturbed at the time of operation. Hysterectomised women report more severe symptoms than women who experience the natural menopause. Women who have had a hysterectomy rely on their symptoms in order to identify their time of menopause. Sometimes in this situation a blood test is done to measure the oestradiol and pituitary FSH (Follicule Stimulating Hormone) level. FSH is produced by the pituitary in order to stimulate the ovaries and to make oestrogen during the normal reproductive cycle. When the ovaries stop producing hormones the pituitary produces more FSH in an attempt to stimulate the ovaries. Despite this the oestradiol level remains low but the FSH level continues to increase. Elevated FSH and low oestradiol levels are seen in post-menopausal women. However, because of the fluctuations in hormone levels during the pre-menopause years through to about three years after the menopause, the absence of this specific hormonal pattern does not mean symptoms are not due to the menopause. Blood tests are helpful when positive but are often misleading and confusing if they do not confirm a post-menopausal state.

> For this reason blood tests done to 'diagnose' menopause are of no value.

Tubal Ligation

There has been some concern as to whether tubal ligation for contraception causes an earlier menopause. Some studies have been published that suggest this may be so, however the majority of medical studies has not shown any association between tubal ligation and the onset of menopause. Tubal ligation is known to lower substantially the risk of ovarian cancer although the reason for this is not known.

Premature menopause

Menopause is premature if it occurs before the age of forty. This happens in about eight per cent of women and it is not completely clear why this happens. Ovulation ceases and the ovaries no longer produce oestradiol and progesterone. However, affected women may have a family history of early menopause as mothers, daughters and sisters all tend to have their menopause at a similar age. Premature ovarian failure may even affect women in their twenties to thirties and in some case this is inherited. Menopause may also occur early in women who have been treated for cancer with either anti-cancer drugs or radiation therapy that has affected the ovaries, or who have experienced other major illnesses.

The facts about the menopause

- Average age in Australian women – 50 years
- Average age in smokers – 48.5 years
- Age at menopause is the same in Europe, Asia and North America

Symptoms of the menopause
Why do they occur?

Oestrogen affects not only the reproductive organs, that is the breasts, ovaries, fallopian tubes, uterus, vagina and vulva, but is also important in the maintenance of other body tissues. Oestrogen acts directly on the skin, heart, lower urinary tract, liver, blood vessels, bone and brain. The major oestrogen produced by the ovaries is oestradiol. So when oestradiol levels suddenly fall, all these body tissues are affected in some way. Interestingly the degree to which different parts of the body are affected and the way in which a woman experiences these changes vary dramatically from individual to individual.

The ovaries and adrenal glands continue to produce variable amounts of weak oestrogens for years after the menopause. Oestrone is the major oestrogen after the menopause. It is produced in fat tissue from hormones produced by the adrenal glands. Women who are more corpulent usually have higher oestrone levels than thin women. The variation in oestrone levels between different women after the menopause is one reason why women experience such variation in menopausal symptoms.

> *There is no uniform experience of the menopause and no single management plan.* Every woman will have her own individual experience and her symptoms can be judged only in the framework of *her personal experience.*

Common manifestations

The symptoms of the menopause are categorised as being physiological,

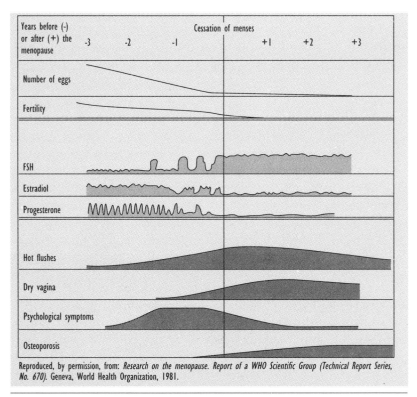

Reproduced, by permission, from: *Research on the menopause. Report of a WHO Scientific Group (Technical Report Series, No. 670).* Geneva, World Health Organization, 1981.

Figure 1. Relationship between hormone changes and symptoms during the menopause transition.

affecting the body systems, or psychological, affecting mood. The psychological changes women have appear to be just as dependent on the fall in oestrogen as the physiological symptoms. In addition, just as psychological experiences are influenced by a woman's immediate environment, so may be the physical symptoms. Therefore, for clarity only, symptoms will be divided into physical and psychological experiences.

Physical changes:
THE FLUSH
Changes in the vascular system result in hot flushes and sweats. No reference to the hot flush has been found in Greek or Roman literature. In 1712 Lawrence Hyster wrote about a German dowager who had lost her periods and experienced intermittent commotion in the blood, characterised by starting in the stomach and accompanied by facial heat and reddening. In Victorian days various remedies were recommended for flushes including baths, shaving the head, not sleeping on a soft mattress and the avoidance of large gatherings. Other treatments also used to control menopausal flushes in the past have included:

enemas	bromide
purgatives	chloral hydrate
phlebotomy	phenobarbitone
hot baths	antidepressants
pelvic diathermy	benzodiazepines

Fortunately society is emerging from these dark days of inappropriate therapy.

> About forty per cent of Australian menopausal women have bothersome hot flushes.

The experience of flushing is very variable, the onset may be pre- or postmenopausal and the duration can be months to years. The intensity and frequency may even vary significantly in the same woman. Some women never have a flush whereas others have devastating symptoms with embarrassingly frequent flushes during the day and sleep deprivation from frequent hot sweats at night. Often women describe shivering episodes following their night sweats and become quite concerned. Flushes are classically aggravated by hot weather, hot drinks, alcohol and stressful situations. Many women are also troubled by a continual or intermittent sensation of being overheated.

Hot flushes do not occur exclusively in women. They also occur in men who have had their testes removed surgically and become deprived of testosterone, the major sex hormone in men.

The exact mechanism of the flush is still unknown. Research indicates that the sensation of excessive heat and the hot flush result from a change in the brain centre for temperature regulation. But oestradiol also affects the constriction and dilation of blood vessels in the skin. Therefore the flush is more complicated than it appears. The menopausal hot flush is totally different to a blush experienced by people of all ages.

- seventeen per cent of regularly menstruating women over the age of forty have hot flushes.
- Five to ten years after menopause thirty-five per cent of women still have hot flushes.

TIREDNESS

As a result of either disturbed sleep from night sweats, or inexplicable insomnia which is not uncommon, unusual tiredness is a frequent complaint of menopausal women. Previously very active and energetic women understandably become quite concerned when they suffer lethargy which compromises their lifestyle. Unexplained headaches are less commonly a troublesome symptom.

SKIN SENSATION

Some women experience a crawling sensation under their skin which usually disappears with oestrogen replacement. Others describe a non-specific change in tactile (touch) sensation such that being touched by others becomes unpleasant. Women should feel reassured that such changes are not uncommon.

JOINT PAINS

Although arthritis is not clearly linked to the menopause, many women develop arthritis-like symptoms with joint and muscle aches. These often resolve with oestrogen treatment.

Urinary Tract

The tissues lining the bladder and urinary passage and the muscles supporting the bladder change when oestradiol levels fall. Therefore urinary frequency and loss of control of urine may occur. The vagina and vulva need oestrogen to remain healthy, and without oestrogen the usual vaginal secretions are not produced. Because of these tissue changes and the vaginal dryness, intercourse may become painful and unpleasant, and the natural resistance to vaginal infections is reduced.

Subsequent urinary problems include:
- Recurrent urinary tract infections
- Urinary incontinence
- Local vaginal discomfort

More than fifty per cent of women aged sixty to sixty-five-have *at least one* of these problems.

Urinary incontinence is under-diagnosed and under-treated despite its far-reaching effects. One out of every eight menopausal women suffers some degree of incontinence and this increases to one in four women in later years! Not only is incontinence embarrassing and uncomfortable but it has a huge negative impact on the quality of life. Women find themselves confined to home, or plan their day around easy access to a toilet. Fear of the embarrassment of urinary incontinence after sex frequently interferes with sexual activity which is very distressing for the affected woman and her partner. Amongst older women, rejection by family members may prematurely precipitate admission to a nursing home —a dire consequence for an often preventable problem.

Acknowledgment of the problem is the first step to seeking help. Many women are embarrassed to speak to their doctor about the problem, possibly because incontinence has such negative associations.

> Physiotherapists can assist women with pelvic floor exercises with success rates of twenty to fifty per cent of patients being cured and sixty per cent of women experiencing overall improvement.

Pelvic floor rehabilitation includes the use of pelvic floor exercises, bladder retraining and other specialised physiotherapy techniques. Adherence to the exercise program is vital to treatment success. Most women do not realise that to really improve or cure the incontinence problem a considerable commitment to do the exercises is required. It is also important to consult a physiotherapist interested and trained in pelvic floor rehabilitation. In some instances, surgery may be necessary.

Oestrogen will help prevent ageing of the urogenital tract and alleviate existing incontinence. Vaginal oestrogen, including low dose therapy that doesn't require additional progesterone, will restore the vaginal lining and normal bacterial levels of lacto bacilli which act as a defence against other infections. This minimises the risk of recurrent thrush and urinary tract infections. Many women also find that local or oral oestrogen therapy reduces urinary urgency, local pain and irritation and night time urinary frequency.

SEXUALITY

The greatest predictive factors for sexual activity and satisfaction after the menopause are the frequency and satisfaction in the preceding years. Women who enjoy pleasurable, active sexual experiences before the menopause are more than likely to continue to do so *with little or no change* in enjoyment, frequency of intercourse or orgasm. Like all potential menopause symptoms, there is much individual variation in sexuality after the menopause. Many women released from the anxiety of pregnancy, with more leisure time, and reduced distraction by their children have enhanced libido, and sexual experience may have a widening place in their lives.

Some pre- and post-menopausal women experience loss of libido which occurs for a variety of reasons. Simple factors such as sleep deprivation from night flushes and vaginal dryness are easily treated.

Vaginal dryness and irritation may make intercourse very uncomfortable and therefore can certainly affect libido. In addition the oestrogen-deficient, less acidic vagina is more prone to infection. The thinning of the vaginal tissues in some women comes on gradually, but in others it can appear quite suddenly. It may occur very rapidly when the ovaries are surgically removed. Some women manage adequately using lubricants such as KY jelly. There are now available a variety of oestrogen preparations that can be used locally within the vagina which reverse these changes without having any oestrogenic effects on the rest of the body. These low dose oestrogen creams or tablets are an important alternative for women who only want to treat these localised symptoms.

Psychological symptoms like irritability, depression and anxiety also contribute to loss of libido. Many women feel a sense of loss and guilt when they become disinterested in sex, and this can further contribute to depressed moods after the menopause. This is often so when they have had a good sexual relationship with their partners. Frequently women also may feel they are becoming less attractive to their partner because of their ageing body. This may be linked to lowered or poor self-esteem.

A number of women find that they cannot stand close physical contact, even with a much-loved partner, and avoid being touched in even non-sexual ways. The classic statement is 'I just can't bear to be touched!' This situation is obviously upsetting to the woman and confusing to her partner, resulting in avoidance of intimate relationships. We do not understand why this disturbance in tactile or touch sensation occurs but it is reasonably common. In both males and females, sexual responsiveness tends to become slower with ageing. Many women become anxious about their slowness to orgasm. If this is openly discussed with the partner, it may be revealed that they too have some concerns regarding their changing sexual prowess. Modifications in sexual technique combined with a relaxed acceptance of one's changing physical responses should result in enhanced sexual enjoyment.

It is normal for the ovaries to produce small amounts of testosterone which is an androgen or virilising hormone and is the major sex hormone in men. Testosterone may be an important factor in maintaining muscle strength and bone density and may contribute to female sexuality in terms of libido and orgasm. After the menopause, particularly after premature or surgical menopause, replacement of small amounts of testosterone may improve sexuality (see chapter 8).

Changes in sexuality cannot be considered without including the partner. Diminished sexual interest or ability may occur in the partner due to stress, or ill health. A change in the nature of the relationship may be the basis for lowered sexuality and always needs to be considered. While sexual intercourse usually improves relationships it is not the only factor. Many couples in their later years find that mutual respect and the shared experiences of surviving the various ups and downs of life produce bonds that perhaps substitute for the loss of sexual experience. It is important that those women who do not have the same sexual desires after menopause that they felt in their youth do not feel they have nothing left to offer their partners, as long relationships usually have so many other positive aspects.

PSYCHOLOGICAL CHANGES

Self-esteem is fundamental for any person to function independently, confidently and happily. A sense of self-worth and enjoyment are essential for optimal quality of life.

Psychological changes around the menopausal years can be very distressing. Most importantly it is now acknowledged that *the psychological effects tend to be maximal before the menopause.* Clearly the fluctuating hormonal levels in the pre-menopause years play a part in this and many women report an escalation of pre-menstrual symptoms in the cycles leading up to their menopause. In addition, life-experiences during this time are important modifiers of these symptoms. Complaints such as fatigue, depression and irritability are common, as are agitation and panic. Many women who have busy, responsible and complicated lives describe being suddenly unable to cope. Women often describe feeling that they don't want to even get up in the morning because they have no idea as to how they are going to get through the day. Everything becomes overwhelming, and the previously organised person is in despair at suddenly being out of control. Women also describe loss of short-term memory and concentration, which not only interferes with their daily activities but may have major effects on their ability to cope in the work place. Difficulty making simple decisions is also experienced by many women. Self-deprecatory feelings of being inadequate, unloved, unattractive and lacking self-esteem may be associated with the already mentioned symptoms, or occur as a symptom alone. Loss of self-esteem is probably the most important of all the feelings mentioned. The effects of past experiences, expectations and environment are fundamental to the way in which each woman psychologically experiences her menopause (see chapter 1).

Research has revealed that up to thirty per cent of women have psychological symptoms related to the menopause and that all improve considerably with oestrogen replacement.

THE BIOLOGICAL BASIS FOR THE PSYCHOLOGICAL SYMPTOMS

Oestrogen is metabolised in the liver and one of its by-products, catechol-oestrogen, has a role in the central nervous system, and may either directly or indirectly modify brain function. Oestrogen may modify thought processes such as concentration and memory, as well as influencing the regions of the brain controlling mood. The presence of any physical symptoms also clearly affect well-being and mood, another reason why the separation of symptoms into psychological and physical is not helpful.

Menopause—the long term effects

The symptoms already discussed occur any time from the pre-menopause years through to several years after the menopause. The so-called long-term effects do not become manifest for many years after the menopause and include osteoporosis and cardiovascular disease. These will be dealt with in detail in separate chapters, however, there are some points to be made concerning both conditions.

> The presence or absence of menopausal symptoms in no way predicts the likelihood of the development of osteoporosis or cardiovascular disease.

The development of osteoporosis and cardiovascular disease depends on multiple factors. The sudden fall in oestradiol levels at menopause is only one factor but an extremely significant one with respect to the development of both conditions. Genetics and lifestyle factors obviously play a major role in the development of these diseases. In the next chapters osteoporosis and cardiovascular disease are discussed mainly in terms of their relationships with the menopause.

Summing up

The list of symptoms associated with the menopause is extensive and each is extremely variable. It cannot be emphasised enough that every woman will have a different experience and similarly will find a therapy suitable for her, be it conventional medication, diet, exercise, counselling, stress management or natural therapy. Just as women's physical and emotional responses to pregnancy and childbirth differ in the extreme, so do their transitions through the menopause. Acknowledgement of these differences and the diversity of experiences should dispel any guilt suffered by those going through a particularly bad menopause and promote support from others around them.

By approaching the menopause with a positive attitude, a healthy lifestyle and equipped with an understanding of her own biology each woman will be able to deal with this transition time the best way possible.

Chapter 3

PREVENTION OF OSTEOPOROSIS: CHILDHOOD THROUGH TO THE LATER YEARS

Bone is made up of living cells in an ever-changing tissue or matrix. The bone cells are constantly remodelling their surrounding tissue by reabsorbing and simultaneously replacing it. When breakdown exceeds replacement then nett bone loss occurs. After maximal bone strength is reached in the years following puberty there are several stable years during which time bone replacement and reabsorption are balanced. From approximately the early forties onwards both men and women slowly lose bone by an age-dependent process in which bone formation is relatively impaired. Bones are made of a dense outer shell, or cortex and an inner woven or trabecular structure. After reaching peak bone strength or density a woman loses on average thirty-five per cent of the outer bone cortex and fifty per cent of the inner woven bone during her lifetime. In contrast, a man would only have approximately two-thirds of this loss. Thus significant bone loss is far more common in women than men because women lose more bone and live longer.

Oestrogen is essential in women for the development of strong, healthy bones during puberty and for the maintenance of strong bones during adult life. When menopause occurs, oestrogen levels fall, directly causing bone loss.

The menopause results in an accelerated phase of bone loss with approximately two per cent of bone being lost each year for the first five or so years after the menopause. This means that as a direct consequence of menopause up to ten per cent of bone is lost from the skeleton in the first five post-menopausal years. The menopausal bone loss occurs in addition to the loss of bone due to ageing, which at this time is minimal in comparison. Lack of oestrogen leads to increased bone breakdown and increased calcium loss in the urine. Bone formation does not increase to compensate for the extra bone breakdown. Oestrogen replacement commenced at the onset of menopause prevents this bone loss. This accelerated loss gradually diminishes until at about ten years after the menopause the continued bone loss is said to be predominantly by the age-dependent mechanism described above. If age-dependent bone loss is independent of oestrogen, then theoretically women on long-term oestrogen should start losing bone again about ten years after the menopause. This does not occur, which indicates that

> all post-menopausal bone loss is in some way hormone dependent even many years after menopause has passed.

Once a critical amount of bone has been lost the condition *osteoporosis* occurs. *'Osteo' means 'bone' and 'porosis' means 'having many small holes'.* The architecture of osteoporotic bone is changed so that the material in which the bone cells lie has many open spaces. Osteoporotic bone is clearly more brittle than normal bone. The importance of osteoporosis arises from the increased risk of fracture which it entails and therefore the diagnosis should only be made when substantial bone loss can be clearly identified (see page 31).

The most common sites of osteoporotic fracture are the wrist, spine (vertebrae) and hip.

- Wrist fractures affect one woman in six and usually result from a fall on an outstretched arm.
- *Spinal crush fractures* may occur in very osteoporotic bone with little or no trauma and result in loss of height, forward curvature of the back (Dowager's hump) and sometimes chronic pain. One in three women over the age of sixty-five experiences a vertebral fracture of this type.
- *Hip fractures* are clinically more severe since this type of fracture is fatal in up to twenty per cent of instances, and of those who survive a hip fracture half will require long-term hospitalisation entailing extended nursing care and loss of independence. This kind of fracture is the most significant result of osteoporosis, both in terms of consequences for the individual and costs to the

community. The health cost of hip fracture alone in dollars to the community is immense, currently being approximately $300 million per year in Australia. Much of this is now preventable.

There is a clear relationship between low bone strength (bone density) and the occurrence of osteoporotic fractures. Some people talk about a 'fracture threshold'; a bone density value above this threshold suggests the risk of fracture is small and a bone density value below the fracture threshold suggests an increased likelihood of fracture. However, the use of the fracture threshold is controversial as in reality bone density measurements are only highly predictive of fracture if they are very low.

There are some important points to be made about 'risk factors' for osteoporosis (discussed later in this chapter) and 'risk factors' in general.

- 'Risk factors' for osteoporosis and osteoporotic fracture have been identified by statistical means with data based on population studies and scientific research on factors affecting bone metabolism. They provide helpful guidelines in terms of recommendations for optimal lifestyle such as diet and exercise, but are of little or no value in identifying the specific individuals who will ultimately develop osteoporosis or sustain a fracture.

- Labelling women 'at risk' may result in asymptomatic well women believing that they already have an established disease. This should not be the case. Risk factors should be used predominantly in preventative medicine in the community as a whole and only applied to the individual in order to prevent a disease, not identify a disease.

- Low bone density indicates *increased risk* of future fracture but such a fracture *does not inevitably* occur. There is considerable overlap in bone density values between women who do and do not sustain fractures.

- A woman who has had one or more vertebral fractures due to osteoporosis in the past is highly likely to have further fractures irrespective of her bone density.

Some further points must be emphasised:
- *The increased tendency of the elderly to fall is a major independent and preventable factor in the occurrence of hip fractures in later life.* Unexpected falls due to simple environmental hazards, unidentified medical problems or medication side-effects are frequently

preventable. Strategies to minimise the likelihood of falls in the elderly are as important as identifying the presence of osteoporosis.

- Once a significant amount of bone has been lost the possible therapies for increasing bone mass are limited and may have undesirable side-effects. Furthermore, *there is no convincing evidence that increasing bone density will prevent future fractures* in women with low bone mass and no prior fractures, although available data indicates this is a reasonable assumption to make.

- Oestrogen replacement is the only treatment proven to *prevent* post-menopausal bone loss and reduce the incidence of osteoporotic fractures.

Clearly the above facts indicate that the way to prevent osteoporotic fractures is to prevent osteoporosis.

Prevention of osteoporosis begins in childhood and can be simplified to three concepts:

1 Attainment of maximal bone strength (bone density)
2 Maintenance of bone density
3 Prevention of bone loss

1 Attainment of maximal bone strength

Until recently it was believed that bone strength peaked in the middle thirties but evidence now suggests that peak bone density may be achieved soon after puberty in the late teens. Sex, race and heredity all exert major influences on bone development.

The bone density of teenage girls reflects their parents' bone densities. Adolescent girls achieve close to their expected peak bone mass by the age of sixteen with only a small increase occurring after this age. This is due to a rapid increase in bone mass during puberty. Sex hormones play an important role in the attainment of peak bone mass at this time.

> Low body weight and low oestradiol levels are associated with lower bone density.

Interestingly, there is a relationship between high dietary fibre, bone density and low oestrogen levels such that female adolescents who have lower than expected bone density associated with low oestrogen tend to consume much more fibre in their diet than their normal counterparts.

This may be due to obsessional dietary behaviour in this sub-group of teenagers. However, a very high fibre diet may decrease calcium absorption as well as reducing oestrogen levels. This is because phytates, which are contained in bran and various vegetables, inhibit the absorption of calcium. Food items high in oxalic acid, such as broccoli, also decrease calcium absorption. This is confusing because broccoli and spinach are listed as good food sources of calcium, but despite their high calcium content, their calcium is poorly absorbed.

Activity during puberty also affects bone development.

Moderate activity probably has little effect on bone mass whereas endurance training in either athletes or dancers is associated with reduced bone mass. Frequently elite athletes and dancers develop *amenorrhoea,* which means they stop ovulating and their periods cease. This is due to the complex interactions between the effect of exercise on the brain, low body weight and, in the case of dancers, a tendency towards anorexia. Loss of periods may occur in athletes, dancers, girls with anorexia nervosa, and several medical conditions. Because of their low oestrogen levels these girls lose bone by a mechanism similar to postmenopausal bone loss.

It is difficult to determine the primary cause of bone loss in this setting but the most important factor appears to be low sex hormone levels, particularly oestrogen but also testosterone, and low body weight.

> Osteoporosis-type fractures may occur in young long distance female runners and women with a long history of anorexia nervosa.

Many believe that young women with irregular or absent menstruation should be given oestrogen replacement, and there is no question that all such girls should discuss this matter with their doctor. Bone loss in adolescents with anorexia nervosa is partly recovered with weight gain even before menstruation resumes. However, even after recovery from anorexia nervosa, bone mass remains below that of other young women and it appears that this deficit persists. *In fact, oestrogen deficiency during adolescence from whatever cause probably results in persistently reduced bone mass.*

Teenagers and young women who go on extreme diets, exercise extensively or who suffer from anorexia nervosa are in danger of experiencing bone fractures when young as well as developing osteoporosis in later life.

Cigarette smoking is common, and increasing in teenagers and young women. We know that smoking is associated with reduced bone mass in later life, but there is no information as to whether the deleterious effect of smoking is possibly enhanced in girls smoking during puberty. Young women who smoke also need to be targeted from a preventative health aspect.

The calcium debate—childhood

Until recently the calcium debate has focused on older women, but now there is greater interest in the diet of our children.

In earlier years the average Australian child's diet had plentiful calcium, especially when all primary school children had milk provided at school recess. Now many children may have inadequate calcium intake for various reasons. One major reason is that the children's diets often reflect their parents' choice of food. Many 'health conscious' families are choosing low-fat, high-fibre diets with little dairy produce. The other extreme is the fast-food-dependent lifestyle with food of high-fat but low nutritional quality. There is however a happy medium and children can have an inexpensive but nutritional diet containing adequate calcium (see Table 2). Young children in most circumstances should drink full cream milk as they require a certain amount of fat for normal growth and development. There is some preliminary evidence that children given added calcium achieve greater bone density more rapidly, however there is no long-term evidence for this.

Meeting the recommended intake of calcium is even a greater problem in adolescents, especially females who do not, for various individual reasons, eat enough calcium.

Young girls frequently adopt diets low in calcium when they try to avoid so called 'fattening foods'. Again, there is no evidence that excessive calcium at this stage alters bone strength, but a minimum intake of 1200 mg daily is needed to maximise bone development. Girls should

Table 1: Risk factors for osteoporosis:

- family history—mother/sister with osteoporosis
- Caucasian/Chinese
- low body mass (below 50 kg)
- tobacco use
- alcohol excess (above 2 standard drinks per day)
- caffeine excess (more than 3 cups of tea/coffee per day)
- chronic poor nutrition
- sedentary lifestyle
- medications
- glucocorticosteroids
- excess thyroxine
- anticoagulants
- disease states
- thyrotoxicosis
- Cushings Syndrome
- Rheumatoid arthritis

be encouraged to eat dairy products and be made aware that there are plenty of low-fat foods with a high calcium content.

The pressure on young girls in Western society to achieve a slim body has far-reaching consequences in terms of physical and psychological health. Transition from the pre-adolescent body to a more voluptuous physique is perceived by many young girls as a disaster. They resent the natural feminine body shape with rounded hips and thighs because it is unfashionable. Their response to the pubertal change is no different to that of their mothers who respond to the menopause and the possibility of HRT with, 'But I don't want to put on weight!' Perhaps women today need to review the work of the great Italian Art Masters and rediscover the beauty of the feminine physique.

Our understanding of the way in which genetically determined peak bone mass can be achieved is incomplete, however some general recommendations can be made:

- Infants and children need to have at least 500 mg calcium per day.
- For adolescents, a diet of at least 1200 mg calcium daily in combination with moderate exercise is optimal.
- Alcohol and cigarettes should be avoided.
- Adolescents and young women with irregular or absent periods should discuss this problem with their doctor in terms of the effect on their bone growth and may need to consider taking oestrogen.

2 Maintenance of bone density

Each individual's genetic make up predetermines many things which may or may not be modified by our environment. Each person's *potential* peak bone density is genetically predetermined, but environmental factors will ultimately affect whether or not this potential is achieved. Therefore, it is important to maximise the benefits that lifestyle and environment can bestow upon bone strength.

After puberty, the next major influences on bone in many women are *pregnancy and lactation.* It is essential that throughout pregnancy, but especially in the third trimester, women increase their calcium intake to meet the combined needs of the foetus and themselves. Also the calcium requirements during lactation are obviously increased, and women often avoid calorie-rich dairy foods when trying to return to their pre-pregnancy weight. Adequate calcium either by diet or supplements, is vital at this time.

Daughters of women with osteoporosis tend to have reduced bone mass. This *hereditary* trend is a significant risk factor for the development of osteoporosis and fracture in daughters of osteoporotic women. A specific genetic marker for low bone density has very recently been identified by Australian scientists. It is hoped that future research may lead to the development of a simple blood test which could be used to identify people at increased risk of osteoporosis. Inheritance has a significant effect on the bone density of various racial groups. Osteoporosis is a relatively common problem amongst Caucasian and Chinese, but less common in Black and Hispanic women. Research has failed to reveal why this is so, but this *racial difference* in osteoporosis and related fractures is not due to diet, timing of puberty or hormonal differences.

Body weight, particularly body fat, is related to bone density in pubertal girls, pre-menopause and post-menopausal women. During puberty, body fat is tightly linked with pubertal maturation and oestrogen production. In later life, fat tissue produces the weak oestrogen called oestrone, which may help prevent bone loss. However body fat appears to influence bone strength by other more significant mechanism(s) not yet fully understood. It is possible that body fat and bone density are genetically linked traits as well. A little corpulence after the menopause is in fact a good thing as far as the bones are concerned.

Lifestyle factors are important in preventing bone loss. *Alcohol* clearly has a bad effect on bone in women, and the extent of this has only

recently been recognised. Chronic alcoholism is a known cause of osteoporosis and high levels of alcohol are toxic to the bone-forming cells.

Women who consume more than two standard drinks of alcohol
per day have significantly reduced bone density.

Women who drink *one to two standard drinks per day* also have lower
bone mass than women who do not drink at all.

Cigarette smoking is particularly bad for bones. Nicotine quite simply
poisons bone cells. It also causes low blood oestrogen levels and this in
turn reduces bone strength.

Physical activity is a major modifier of bone mass, particularly in post-
menopausal women. Activity increases bone mass, and inactivity
decreases it. Several studies have shown that patients lose calcium from
their bones when confined to bed, and this loss continues until the
patients are fully up and about. The clearest example of these effects of
inactivity on bone is the predicament of astronauts exposed to
prolonged weightlessness. Astronauts lose calcium rapidly during space
expeditions when they are in a gravity-free environment. Calcium loss
from the skeleton during extended space flights persists despite special
exercises performed during the flights. It is unclear how this gravita-
tional weight effect transfers into bone metabolism, however *weight-
bearing activity is undoubtedly a vital mechanical stimulus which helps
maintain the balance between bone production and bone breakdown.*

The best exercise for bones involves active weight-bearing movement
such as jogging or walking, or at least vigorous muscle-pull on bone.
Swimming is terrific for cardiovascular fitness and maintaining muscle
strength and flexibility but does not prevent bone loss. The bones have
to get the message that they are carrying the body's weight around for
an exercise to be directly beneficial and help prevent bone loss.

It has been shown that moderate weight-bearing exercise may delay
vertebral bone loss in post-menopausal women. This is in contrast to
the effects of extreme exercise and the risk of low bone density in
athletes whose periods cease!

How much exercise is required to be moderate and effective but not
excessive? *Thirty minutes of weight-bearing exercise three to five times each
week* is probably a good target for most women. A regular program is
essential, and to be effective she needs to place exercise reasonably high

on the list of priorities, and consciously to set aside the time to do it. This does not mean setting unrealistic aims. Jogging around the streets at 6.00 am in the cold is not for everyone. To quote Dr Jean Hailes, '*This is boring. You only have to look at the faces of the people doing it.*' Practical alternatives include walking, tennis, golf, get-fit classes, gardening or anything that keeps you active on your feet. Again, regarding exercise, Jean Hailes said, 'Don't be put off just because it is bad weather; a true saying is that there is no bad weather, only bad clothes for it—buy a good jumper.'

Excessive caffeine intake may be detrimental in terms of calcium balance, but probably only in women with a poor calcium intake. Tea as well as coffee is a major source of caffeine, with the average cup of tea containing as much caffeine as the average up of instant coffee (65—85 mg). Caffeine interferes with the way calcium is handled in the body. It doesn't actually decrease calcium absorption. Therefore the calcium contained in milk coffee such as a cappuccino is still absorbed. However the high caffeine content of cappuccino coffee makes it a less desirable way to obtain calcium.

How much caffeine is too much? It is well documented that people who drink *three or more cups* of tea or coffee daily will experience at least mild withdrawal symptoms when they cease, including fatigue, headaches and irritability. The severity of these symptoms obviously increases in proportion to the amount of caffeine they usually have, with large consumers, five cups a day or more, experiencing severe headache, gastrointestinal symptoms and depression on ceasing.

Several *medications* are related to osteoporosis, the most common being thyroid hormone (thyroxine) and prednisolone, a glucocorticosteroid. Thyroxine is taken by people with an absent or under-active thyroid gland. It is important that the replacement dose is correct, as too much thyroxine stimulates bone turnover and nett bone loss results. The thyroxine level can easily be monitored with simple blood tests. Various severe diseases such as rheumatoid arthritis, asthma and lupus frequently require treatment with prednisolone. Prolonged therapy may result in considerable bone loss and so it is best for treatment to be of the minimal effective dose for the briefest possible time. Some people require chronic prednisolone therapy, and in such instances attention to calcium intake and weight-bearing exercise is paramount. Combined therapy with calcitriol (Vitamin D3) and calcium may also limit bone loss in women on long-term prednisolone and this aspect should be discussed with the doctors involved.

Acute and chronic diseases as listed in Table 1 are associated with bone loss, and subsequent osteoporosis. Any chronic disease resulting in malabsorption of calcium also has osteoporosis as a possible consequence.

How sensitive are these 'risk' factors in identifying an individual at increased risk of future fracture? As already mentioned risk factors are helpful but individually of limited value.

> The only way to ascertain whether there is an increased likelihood of future osteoporotic fracture in a woman is by direct measurement of her bone density.

Measuring bone density

Bone strength is quantitatively assessed by measuring bone density. Such measurements tell nothing about the quality of the bone present, which

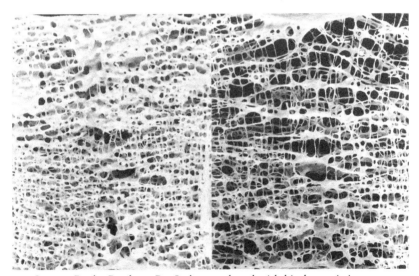

Source: Roche Products Pty Ltd, reproduced with kind permission

Figure 2. Photograph showing normal bone with very small spaces and osteoporotic bone with gaping holes in the bone structure.

is an important determinant of bone strength. As there is no simple clinical way of measuring bone quality, we depend on the assessment of bone density as the primary indicator of bone strength. There are technically several ways by which bone density can be measured and these include single and dual photon absorptiometry, quantitative CT scanning and dual energy x-ray absorptiometry. The latter, commonly known as *DEXA,* is safe, simple, quick, precise and accurate with the patient lying comfortably on an examination couch during the assessment. The machine measures the mineral density of bone which essentially is the amount of calcium salt present in a specific amount of bone. Using DEXA, bone density can be measured at the most important sites of fracture in post-menopausal women, the hip and spine.

As for any medical test, bone density measurements should only be done if the result will affect patient management or therapy. To randomly screen large numbers of women by bone densimetry is both costly and inappropriate.

There is no value in measuring bone density in a woman who has already decided on hormone replacement as the result will not alter her management. Alternatively the knowledge of a woman's bone density may be a major factor in her decision regarding HRT.

Bone density measurements are also used to monitor possible bone loss in higher risk individuals, assess the severity of osteoporosis and monitor the response to treatment in women with established osteoporosis.

3 Preventing bone loss

Calcium—before the menopause

During the reproductive years, excluding pregnancy and lactation, regularly menstruating women have continuous oestrogen production by their ovaries. Providing an adequate calcium intake is maintained, there appears to be no benefit from further calcium supplementation.

There is some evidence that the calcium regulatory hormones can adjust to low calcium intakes and that the body can be relatively effective in conserving calcium. However with extremely low calcium intakes (below 200 mg daily) the body ultimately loses calcium with mobilisation of calcium from bone and thus bone loss. The optimal situation is to consume sufficient dietary calcium to keep the body calcium levels in balance. The present recommended daily amount for pre-menopause women in developed countries is 800 mg per day, however many agree this is an underestimate, and most women would be better off consuming closer to 1200 mg per day.

In less developed countries women appear to maintain bone strength with lower calcium intakes, however overall life style factors such as different food content of their diet, abstinence from alcohol, caffeine and nicotine and possibly greater physical activity all interact to create this difference.

The primary dietary source of calcium is dairy produce. Milk is an excellent calcium-containing food and even full cream milk is relatively low in fat (see Table 2). The fat content of full cream milk is only 3.9 per cent, calcium enriched milk 1.2 per cent and skim milk 0.1 per cent. Some soya milk products have added calcium, however many available soya milks have high salt and aluminium contents and are not an ideal long-term alternative. Anyone using soya milk as a calcium source should find out how much aluminium and salt is in the brand they are using—it may be necessary to contact the manufacturer for this information.

Multiple dairy food alternatives exist, with the extensive varieties of cheeses and yoghurts displaying both the energy and calcium content on their packaging. The only truly valuable non-dairy source of calcium in the diet is tinned fish such as sardines and salmon. The calcium-rich component of these fish is in their bones which need to be eaten in order to get the calcium.

High protein diets may alter calcium balance depending on the specific proteins consumed but most natural proteins such as meat do not increase calcium loss. Long-term use of aluminium-containing antacids may lead to calcium loss and bone reabsorption and their chronic use should be avoided.

CALCIUM IN PREGNANCY AND LACTATION

For normal intra-uterine growth the foetus requires calcium, and the mother must supply it. Although most of the calcium is taken up by the foetus in the last three months of pregnancy, pregnant women have enhanced calcium absorption from their diet from the beginning of pregnancy. However it has been calculated that one-third of the calcium needs of the foetus comes from the mother's skeleton. Therefore the daily calcium intake during pregnancy should be at least 1000 mg, but preferably closer to

2000 mg. If this cannot be achieved by diet, then calcium supplements should be taken. Again, throughout breast-feeding there is substantial maternal calcium loss through the milk and an intake close to 2000 mg daily either through diet or supplements is appropriate to prevent bone loss.

CALCIUM—MENOPAUSE AND BEYOND

Calcium requirements are higher in post-menopausal women, possibly due to decreased intestinal absorption of calcium with age combined with increased loss of calcium in the urine. Low oestrogen levels after the menopause lead to bone breakdown and the calcium lost from this bone is excreted from the body in the urine. Oestrogen replacement therapy stops bone breakdown and calcium loss.

Since 1988, over forty-three studies have been published in which the relationship between calcium intake and bone strength have been investigated. More than half of these identified a positive link between calcium intake and bone strength, but one-third did not. Clearly the role of calcium in preventing osteoporosis is still controversial.

> In the first five years after menopause, the underlying cause of bone loss is oestrogen withdrawal, with calcium intake being of relatively little significance.

> Calcium supplementation within the first five post-menopausal years is of little or no use in preventing bone loss.

Calcium supplementation appears to positively retard bone loss in women five or more years post-menopause who consume low calcium diets. There is unfortunately some confusion as to the amount of calcium 'low' represents, however a diet of less than 400 mg of calcium daily can be safely declared low. The next issue is how much calcium is required? Again, for various reasons the extensive research data available does not produce a consistent figure. A calcium intake of 1500 mg daily is recommended for post-menopausal women, as this is the average requirement to maintain overall calcium balance. This is probably two to three times that consumed by the average Australian post-menopausal woman. There is no reason why older post-menopausal women should not take calcium supplements if their diet remains low in calcium for whatever reason. Calcium tablets have no side-effects, particularly there is no evidence that increasing dietary calcium causes kidney stones, in fact recent evidence suggests the reverse.

Various forms of calcium supplements are available from chemists, health food shops and supermarkets. The *elemental calcium content* of the supplement should be clearly indicated on the container, and equals the amount of *available* calcium in each tablet. Calcium absorption, has been shown to be greater if the calcium is taken in divided doses during the day and at night. *Citric acid* (found in orange juice) also improves calcium absorption. *Calcium citrate* is an excellent form of supplement, but commercial availability is limited. Alternatively other compounds such as calcium gluconate, lactate or carbonate can be used and taken with orange juice. Women often find they prefer one calcium preparation to another. Effervescent tablets contain about 400 mg of sodium (common salt). The safe intake of sodium daily is 900—2000 mg and the effervescent supplements make up a considerable percentage of the daily salt allowance, and are not ideal for women on salt-restricted diets. Some calcium supplements contain dolomite, or bone meal which is high in calcium but still controversial as a calcium supplement as it has been reported that this calcium compound contains lead.

Summary

- In the early post-menopausal years, calcium intake needs to be adequate, at least 800 mg daily, but there is no evidence that further supplementation prevents bone loss.
- Women five or more years post-menopause not taking oestrogen should have a calcium intake of 1200—1500 mg daily, but there is no evidence of any benefit of a calcium intake above this.
- Post-menopausal women taking oestrogen have the same calcium requirements as pre-menopause women.

The role of hormones

The only proven effective therapy for the preventation and management of oestrogen-related bone loss is oestrogen.

This applies not only to post-menopausal women, but also to younger women whose ovaries produce insufficient oestrogen to protect their bones (see p. 25).

By acting directly on bone cells via specific oestrogen receptors, oestrogen prevents bone breakdown (reabsorption). If oestrogen replacement is begun close to menopause, the early phase of post-menopausal bone loss is prevented. However this effect is maintained only whilst oestrogen is taken, once oestrogen is ceased post-menopausal bone loss ensues. Therefore anyone who decides to take oestrogen specifically to prevent bone loss really needs to take it long-term in order to gain the true benefits. This means for at least ten years. Long-term oestrogen not only prevents bone loss, but more significantly reduces the likelihood of osteoporotic fractures of the spine and hip.

If commenced six or more years after the menopause, oestrogen results in an initial increase in bone mass of about five per cent in the first year, and stops further bone loss. The increase in bone density observed in women starting oestrogen several years after their menopause also occurs if osteoporosis is already established. In women with osteoporosis, oestrogen has been shown to reduce the likelihood of vertebral fracture by up to fifty per cent. It is never too late to commence oestrogen as the beneficial effects on bone are seen even in elderly women.

The overall risks and benefits of oestrogen should be considered by each woman. Clearly women reaching the menopause with low bone mass and increased risk of osteoporosis and fracture should seriously think about using it. Alternatively women with normal or greater bone mass may have little to gain, in terms of ultimately preventing fracture, by taking oestrogen. Some women enter the menopause with normal or high bone density but then go on to lose bone at a faster rate than others. We cannot predict who is likely to be a 'fast loser' of bone. Therefore women who choose not to take oestrogen on the basis of their adequate bone density measurement, should have their bone density remeasured eighteen to twenty-four months later to be sure they are not losing bone at an unacceptable rate.

Women with a past or current history of breast cancer frequently express concern that they are destined to lose bone and they are advised against taking oestrogen. Two potential alternatives deserve consideration: progestogens and tamoxifen. Progestogens may prevent bone loss to some extent, however the evidence to support this is incomplete. Progestogens are not recommended for the treatment of osteoporosis. Tamoxifen is a synthetic drug that acts as an anti-oestrogen, and is commonly used in the management of breast cancer. Recent studies have shown that tamoxifen prevents post-menopausal bone loss, although it is not yet known whether long-term tamoxifen prevents osteoporotic fractures. There are now some long-term studies under way which will evaluate the effect of tamoxifen in preventing bone loss and fractures.

Osteoporosis—other therapies

All treatment strategies for established osteoporosis should include adequate calcium intake as discussed earlier and, wherever possible, weight-bearing exercise. When the possibility of weight-bearing exercise is limited, exercise in water will improve flexibility and muscle strength and enhance overall health and well-being. Prolonged bed rest only accelerates bone loss and should be avoided.

Oestrogen will improve bone mass by about five per cent in women with osteoporosis, and prevent further bone loss and fracture. The efficiency of other therapies is less well documented, and many of the newer agents are associated with problematic side-effects. Only a brief comment is made about these other medications here, as further detail is beyond the scope of this book.

Calcitonin is a hormone produced by the thyroid gland. Calcitonin has been shown to prevent bone loss in the peri- and early post-menopausal years and in patients with osteoporosis. Whether therapy actually reduces fracture rate is yet to be established.

Calcitriol is 1,25-dihydroxyvitamin D3, the principal active form of vitamin D. Calcitriol stimulates calcium absorption from the diet and may prevent bone reabsorption and perhaps increase bone formation. A combination of calcitriol and calcium may prevent hip and vertebral fractures, however there are concerns that widespread use of calcitriol and other vitamin D supplements may result in side-effects such as high blood and urine calcium levels and kidney stones. Vitamin D supplements should only be taken with careful medical supervision.

Anabolic steroids: This group of drugs are androgens, meaning they act on the male hormone receptor, and when given in very high doses result in masculinising side-effects. Nandrolone decanoate may increase spinal bone density over twelve to eighteen months. Many

Table 2 Foods rich in calcium

Food	Calcium Content	Food	Calcium Content
Dairy Foods		Nuts	
Milk:		Almonds, 50 g	125 mg
Full cream, 1 cup	300 mg	Brazil, 50 g	90 mg
Skinny, 1 cup	383 mg	Peanuts, 50 g	30 mg
Rev, 1 cup	375 mg	Grains & Cereals	
Big M, 1 cup	295 mg	Bran Flakes, 30 g	20 mg
Yoghurt, 200 g	300 mg	Bread, 1 slice	15 mg
Cheese-Cheddar, 1 slice	300 mg	Meat	
Cottage cheese, 200 g	190 mg	Red or white, av. serve	15 mg
Fish		Sausage, 2 grilled	84 mg
Sardines (with bones) 100 g	300 mg	Beefburger, fried, 60 g	30 mg
Salmon (with bones) 100 g	300 mg	Miscellaneous	
Oysters, 12 only	230 mg	Pizza with cheese, 150 g	240 mg
Vegetables		Quiche Lorraine, 150 g	260 mg
Broccoli, 100 g	70 mg	Egg, 1 only	30 mg
Pumpkin, 100 g	40 mg	Pasta, 150 g	10 mg
Potatoes, 120 g	10 mg	Sesame seeds (black) 1 tbspn	200 mg
Fruit		Tahine, 20 g	50 mg
Banana, 1 only average	7 mg	Beverages	
Apple, 1 only	9 mg	Ovaltine, 10 g	250 mg
Orange, 1 only	45 mg	Orange juice, 120 g	10 mg
Lemon, 1 only	110 mg	Coffee, percolated, 230 g	2 mg
Dried Figs, 2 only	60 mg	Tea, 230 g	0 mg
Soy Products			
Soy Milk, 250 ml	290 mg		
Soy/Kidney beans, 50 g	70 mg		

patients report reduced pain and increased well-being, and when used as recommended, side-effects are uncommon. Testosterone implants also increase bone density of the hip and spine in both normal women and those with low bone mass. However there is still no proof that increasing bone density actually prevents fractures.

Biphosphonates: These drugs are used to treat Paget's disease and recently have been shown to be effective in osteoporosis. There are a number of different biphosphonates with varying potency and side-effects, and at this stage their long-term safety and efficiency requires further study.

Fluoride: Fluoride is used in several European countries to treat osteoporosis. Fluoride increases bone mass, however it appears the quality of the new bone is not as good as that of normal bone, and the side-effects are considerable. Fluoride is not recommended for routine treatment for these reasons.

Summary

There is currently no ideal medical therapy available to treat osteoporosis. Clearly the key to the problem is prevention.

Prevention involves:

- Attention to *diet* with adequate calcium intake from infancy to old age
- *Weight-bearing exercise*
- *Fall prevention* for those at risk of fracture
- *Consideration of oestrogen therapy* at menopause

Chapter 4

PREVENTION OF CARDIOVASCULAR DISEASE

Heart disease is now the major cause of death in Australian women. The importance of cardiovascular disease as a cause of death in females has doubled from 1921 to the present day, largely as a result of much lower numbers of female deaths from other causes. With the increased life expectancy of Australian women, now eighty years, the impact of heart disease and stroke, not only on mortality, but also on chronic disability is of major concern. Women live longer than men, but experience more years of physical handicap (the average is fourteen years) and on average six of these years are of severe handicap due to ill health—double that of men. There doesn't appear to be much point living longer if the quality of life is poor!

Among post-menopausal women the leading cause of death is coronary artery disease. A fifty year old Caucasian women has a forty-six per cent lifelong chance of developing and a thirty-one per cent chance of dying of heart disease. Again the way to combat this problem is through *prevention.* Primary prevention of heart disease and stroke in women should reduce deaths from heart disease and stroke, but more importantly increase the number of healthy years of expected new life, and therefore the quality of life for many women.

What is cardiovascular disease?

Cardiovascular disease includes disease of the major arteries to the heart, the coronary arteries, the carotid arteries to the brain and the other major arteries supplying the rest of the body. In this chapter only cardiovascular disease due to atherosclerosis will be discussed. Atherosclerosis occurs when the lining of a major artery is injured and fatty deposits build up resulting in the narrowing of the artery. This process is very gradual, occurring over several decades.

Injury to the arteries may be caused by:
- untreated high blood pressure (hypertension)
- smoking tobacco
- high concentrations of cholesterol
- high blood glucose levels (diabetes)
- changes with ageing

The fatty (cholesterol) deposits in the arteries initially appear as yellow streaks, but over years they enlarge—at this stage the term *atherosclerotic plaque* describes the fat deposits. When an atherosclerotic plaque becomes sufficiently large it causes narrowing of the artery and limits blood flow through the artery. When such narrowing exists in the coronary arteries (the main arteries to the heart muscle) chest pain, called angina, occurs because not enough blood is reaching the heart muscle through the narrowed artery. A heart attack (myocardial infarction) occurs when the artery becomes very narrowed, or blocked, and a region of heart muscle dies. The same process can occur in the carotid arteries to the brain, resulting in a stroke, and of course in any other major arteries in the body.

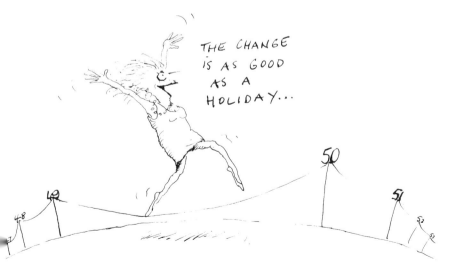

Standard risk factors for atherosclerosis

The major *treatable* factors which cause atherosclerosis and heart disease in women are:

- smoking
- hypertension
- high cholesterol
- obesity
- diabetes mellitus

Of these smoking is by far the most significant. *A strong family history of heart disease is an equally important risk factor.*

Identified risk factors for strokes in women include

- smoking
- high blood pressure
- high cholesterol

Correcting any of the reversible risk factors will significantly reduce the chance of developing cardiovascular disease.

Practically this means:

- long term control of blood pressure
- weight reduction
- giving up smoking
- dietary changes

These are the obvious strategies, and will not be discussed further in this book. Instead I shall focus on the relationship between menopause and cardiovascular disease, and the effects of hormone replacement therapy.

Menopause and heart disease

Women tend to develop cardiovascular disease later in life than men, and at a slower rate. The increased number of deaths due to heart disease in women versus men also reflects the greater number of older women. Natural menopause is probably linked with an increase in cardiovascular disease, although this has not been statistically confirmed. In contrast, surgical menopause (removal of both ovaries) doubles the risk of heart disease, and the use of oestrogen by women with a surgical menopause removes this increased risk. Because surgical menopause results in an acute oestrogen loss, it is easy to demonstrate a clear relationship between it and heart disease. Natural menopause is associated with a very gradual reduction in oestrogen over several years. Therefore any distinct relationship between reduced oestrogen levels and heart disease becomes diluted over time and merges in with the effect of ageing per se, making an association between the two difficult to demonstrate statistically.

Oestrogen replacement therapy and heart disease

Multiple studies have been conducted and data published on the effects of oestrogen on heart disease. These studies consistently demonstrate post-menopausal oestrogen replacement therapy reduces the risk of cardiovascular disease by thirty to fifty per cent.

This protective effect of oestrogen includes healthy post-menopausal women with no risk factors for heart disease, but more importantly *women who have the greatest risk for cardiovascular disease appear to have the greatest benefit.* Oestrogen replacement appears to reduce significantly the likelihood of future cardiovascular disease in women who have hypertension, obesity or are smokers. As already stated, smoking is probably the most important single risk factor for cardiovascular disease in women. Post-menopausal oestrogen use appears to reduce the risk of cardiovascular disease in smokers to that of non-smokers who do not take oestrogen.

What about women who already have cardiovascular disease?

In the past, having angina or a previous heart attack were considered contraindications to HRT. The reverse now applies, and *the greatest benefits of oestrogen replacement are seen in women with known coronary artery narrowing.* The major studies of post-menopausal women with known cardiovascular disease have shown greatly improved life expectancy in women who take oestrogen, compared to women who do not.

The protective effects of oestrogen described above have been observed in multiple controlled long-term studies and are extremely unlikely to be due to any confounding factors. These benefits are consistent with the cholesterol-lowering effects of oestrogen seen in post-menopausal women. It is believed that the cholesterol-lowering effect of oestrogen accounts for about thirty per cent of its overall cardiovascular protection. There are several other ways oestrogen prevents heart disease and exerts its protective effect:

- oestrogen causes widening of the coronary arteries and therefore increased blood flow to the heart;
- oestrogen may prevent thrombosis (blood clotting) in the coronary arteries; and
- oestrogen has directly favourable effects on the function of the cells lining the major arteries, causing a reduction in the build-up of cholesterol deposits in the artery walls.

Importantly this protective effect of oestrogen is seen very soon after oestrogen is commenced, and current users (as opposed to past users) have the greatest benefit. The early onset of the protective effects of oestrogen once it is commenced after menopause is probably due to the immediate direct action oestrogen has on the major arteries.

Oestrogen and stroke

Oestrogen therapy increases blood flow to the carotid arteries to the brain and probably reduces build up of cholesterol deposits in these arteries as in other major arteries. Oestrogen replacement therapy decreases the incidence of stroke and death due to stroke in post-menopausal women who are at increased risk of such events.

Most of the information regarding oestrogen and cardiovascular disease comes from women taking oestrogen only. There are concerns that progesterone may negate the benefits of oestrogen. However animal studies and recent English data show the same reduction in risk for both coronary artery disease and stroke in women taking combined oestrogen and progesterone therapy as seen in women taking oestrogen alone. The fear that progesterone may decrease the benefits of oestrogen has probably been unreasonably overstated. More information on the cardiovascular effects of combined oestrogen and progesterone therapy is required.

Oestrogen replacement therapy and blood fats

Blood fats (lipoproteins) represent a complex and dynamic system by which various forms of fat are stored in and transferred between different cells of the body. There are many subclasses and sub-fractions but the ones routinely measured include total cholesterol and triglycerides. The role of triglycerides in cardiovascular disease is controversial, whereas the importance of cholesterol is well known. The main subclasses of cholesterol relevant to this overview are LDL (low density) cholesterol and HDL (high density) cholesterol.

LDL cholesterol ultimately resulting in the development of athero-sclerosis and high blood levels is of concern.

In contrast, high levels of *HDL cholesterol* are associated with *reduced risk of cardiovascular disease* and are desirable.

When total cholesterol is found to be elevated above normal, further tests should be done to determine whether this is due to increased HDL or LDL cholesterol. If there is elevated HDL cholesterol but normal LDL cholesterol one can be reassured. If the problem is high LDL cholesterol then it is appropriate to try to lower this level. Ideally, the cholesterol level should be reduced by diet, exercise, weight reduction and cessation of smoking. Occasionally special cholesterol-lowering medications are required but these are expensive and may have consider-able side-effects. Oestrogen, even when taken in combination with progesterone, will reduce LDL cholesterol and increase HDL cholesterol (which is desirable). In post-menopausal women, HRT should be considered and perhaps used as a cholesterol-lowering medication as the first alternative.

Current recommendations re HRT and cardiovascular disease in menopausal/post menopausal women:

- Women with low risk of cardiovascular disease—prevention of cardiovascular disease alone is not sufficient reason to recommend HRT.
- Women at high risk or with known cardiovascular disease—HRT should be considered, particularly for women with angina, past heart attacks and/or elevated cholesterol.

Chapter 5

CANCER IN WOMEN

Cancer is predominantly a disease of the older person with fifty-six per cent of all cancers occurring in people over the age of sixty-four. Therefore with our ageing population the incidence of cancers is likely to increase progressively. Overall, cancer is more common in men than women, however, assuming death due to some other cause does not occur earlier than life expectancy, the lifetime risk of developing a cancer in Australian women is one in four. Heart disease remains the major cause of death but cancer is the second most common cause of death in Australia today. Statistics from the Victorian Cancer Registry 1989 Statistical Report, published in 1992 by the Anti-Cancer Council of Victoria, tell us the most common cancer in women is breast cancer followed by cancer of the colon, melanoma, lung, rectal, uterine, ovarian and cervical cancer. However, mortality is greatest for breast cancer, followed by cancer of the colon, lung, pancreas, ovary and stomach. Clearly less common cancers such as pancreas and stomach cancer are more lethal. In order to prevent cancer, we need to focus on the known factors which cause it.

Cancer of the Colon

This is the second most common cancer and cause of cancer death in women. This cancer is almost unheard of in underdeveloped countries such as Africa. Diet plays a vital role in the development of colonic cancer with high-fibre, low-fat and modest protein-containing diets throughout life being the most protective. Most Australian diets, particularly those of children, are low in fibre and excessively high in fat and protein. Interestingly, oestrogen replacement therapy after menopause appears to reduce the risk of bowel cancer by up to forty-five per cent. Preliminary data also indicates that people who regularly use low dose aspirin and other anti-inflammatory medications (not paracetamol) are at decreased risk of bowel cancer. Having a family history of bowel cancer significantly increases your risk of developing this disease. It is strongly recommended that people who have had a parent or sibling with cancer of the colon should have a test called a 'colonoscopy' done after the age of forty and at intervals as low as every five years after that.

Melanoma

Melanoma, a specific form of skin cancer, is being diagnosed more commonly and earlier these days. Limiting sun exposure by staying out of the sun, especially during the peak intensity hours in the middle of the day, wearing protective clothing and high strength sun screens help prevent melanoma and other skin cancers.

Lung Cancer

Lung cancer has increased in women over the last few decades since it became fashionable for women to smoke cigarettes. Most lung malignancies can be prevented if people stop smoking.

The specific cancers which only affect women occur in the cervix, ovary and endometrium. Cancer of the cervix and ovary are discussed in detail in this chapter and cancer of the endometrium is included in the chapter on vaginal bleeding (chapter 6). Breast cancer is not exclusively a cancer of women, although it is exceedingly rare in men. There are some families who appear to be genetically predisposed to breast cancer and in these families the men may also be affected. This, however, is very rare. There are also some uncommon genetic conditions in men which are associated with increased breast cancer risk, the most common of these being Klinefelter's syndrome, which affects the testes and causes male infertility.

In consideration of cancer in general the most important concept to teach and practice is *prevention*. Examples of preventative measures have already been given above. Equally important is *early detection,* because the earlier any cancer can be diagnosed the better the outcome or prognosis. The increasing availability of screening programs including Pap smear and mammography screening, as well as more focused examinations (such as colonoscopy) for people at high risk of other cancers are effective in the early detection of cancer.

Prevention, by modification of diet and lifestyle and early detection of cancer by screening should be incorporated into everyone's life as strategies for healthy living.

The remainder of this chapter focuses on the specific female cancers, including breast cancer, and what can be done in terms of their prevention and detection.

Cancer of the cervix

The lower part of the uterus which is somewhat barrel-shaped and opens into the vagina is known as the *cervix.* Cancer of the cervix is the eighth most common cancer in Australian women, with each woman having a risk of one in one hundred of developing cervical cancer during her lifetime. The most important fact about this cancer is that *cancer of the cervix is highly preventable* by women having a regular medical examination known as a *Pap smear test.*

Cervical cancer occurs most commonly in women aged between fifty-five and sixty. Unfortunately this is not widely recognised and there is a misconception that Pap smear tests are not necessary after the menopause. As few as thirteen per cent of women over the age of fifty-five have regular Pap smear tests—yet this is the group of women in whom cervical cancer is likely to occur! Identification of early changes or pre-cancerous changes in the cells of the cervix can enable treatment which will prevent cancer developing. Even if an early cancer does develop however, early detection by a Pap smear test results in cure in ninety-five per cent of the affected women. Yet in Australia approximately three hundred and fifty women die of cervical cancer each year—these are potentially all preventable deaths.

WHAT IS A PAP SMEAR TEST?

This test is named after Dr Papanicolaou, the person who devised this specific test for cervical cancer. This is a *screening test* which detects abnormal changes in the cells of the cervix. An abnormal result may indicate further investigations are required, depending on the type of abnormality found.

The Pap smear test simply involves the collection of a sample of cells from the cervix and their examination under a microscope by specially trained pathology staff.

Every sexually active woman should have a vaginal examination including a Pap smear test every two years. This should continue at least until the age of seventy after which the necessity for further tests should be discussed by each woman with her doctor. The Royal Australian College of Obstetricians and Gynaecologists generally recommend that women over the age of seventy years who have had a *normal Pap smear test in the preceding five years no longer need to continue to have further Pap smear tests.* If abnormal cells have not been found with a Pap smear test by this age there is little chance of them developing.

A Pap smear test can be performed by either a doctor or nurse trained in the procedure. Many women avoid the examination but, if performed in a comfortable setting, any embarrassment and discomfort should be minimal. The cervix is seen using an instrument called a speculum which, after being warmed and lubricated with water, is inserted into the vagina. With the speculum in place a wooden spatula and a soft brush are used to scrape a sample of cells from the surface of the cervix. These are then transferred onto a glass microscope slide and sent to a specialised laboratory for assessment under the microscope. Uncommonly, the scraping may result in some superficial bleeding which is noticed as light spotting. The result of the Pap smear is usually available within one or two weeks. A normal result indicates the next test should be performed after another two years.

An *abnormal result* has various levels of significance and *does not automatically mean a woman has cancer.* The most common cause of an abnormal result is the presence of a wart virus infection caused by the human papilloma virus. This viral infection is common and usually sexually transmitted. Most women are unaware that they have wart virus infection and are asymptomatic. Less commonly, the virus causes genital warts which can be uncomfortable. More importantly, human papilloma virus infection may cause abnormal changes in the cells of the cervix known as *dysplasia.* Dysplasia may develop without wart virus infection and in itself is not actually cancer, but if left untreated over time will usually progress to cervical cancer. Therefore dysplasia means abnormal changes in the cells of the cervix that occur before cancer of the cervix actually develops. Dysplasia most commonly occurs in women between the ages of twenty and thirty-five years. When diagnosed on a smear test dysplasia is usually described as being mild, moderate or severe. The finding of dysplasia requires further medical assessment by a gynaecologist who can perform a *colposcopy*. A colposcopy is like a more complicated smear test. The cervix can be seen by the gynaecologist in greater detail using special magnification. Small tissue samples are taken from any suspicious areas seen during the colposcopy for further laboratory testing. Again, although not a particularly elegant procedure, colposcopy causes minimal discomfort, does not require an anaesthetic and usually only takes about fifteen minutes to perform.

Dysplasia needs to be treated to stop it changing further into cervical cancer. Localised areas of dysplasia are treated by either diathermy (local heat), laser treatment or by freezing. More extensive or advanced dysplasia may need to be treated by a procedure called a cone biopsy which involves removal of part of the cervix. This requires a general anaesthetic. When the abnormality has progressed to early cervical cancer a hysterectomy is necessary. The most important message is that regular smear tests result in early detection of minor abnormalities which if dealt with immediately do not progress to cancer.

Women who do not have regular smear tests run the risk of having undiagnosed abnormalities progressing to cancerous growths without any symptoms or warning signs of the changes that are occurring.

Pap Test Registry

It is easy to forget when the next Pap smear test is due—many women remember by having their examination on each alternate birthday! In some Australian states a Pap Test Registry has been established and a reminder notice is sent out when a woman's next test is due. This is a voluntary registry which many women find useful. Following any abnormal result, more frequent tests are initially required and appropriately timed reminders are sent out.

Pap smear tests after Hysterectomy

A total hysterectomy involves removal of the body of the uterus as well as the cervix, or mouth of the uterus. Thus cervical cancer will not develop following a standard hysterectomy and regular Pap smears are not needed. The only situation in which this is not the case is in women who have had a hysterectomy for either cervical or endometrial cancer. These women need to continue to have Pap smear tests taken from the top of the vagina to check that abnormal cells have not recurred later in life. Occasionally a sub-total hysterectomy is performed in which the upper part of the uterus is removed and the cervix is left communicating with the vagina. In this instance Pap smears are still needed every two years as the potential for cancer of the cervix to develop still exists.

Ovarian Cancer

The ovaries are the major source of the various female sex hormones through the reproductive years. The immature female eggs are also stored in the ovaries and during each reproductive cycle an egg matures within the ovary before it is expelled into the fallopian tube at ovulation. Therefore the ovaries are made up of several different cell types and each has various functions. Ovarian tumours develop most commonly from the cells on the surface of the ovary. There are several different types of ovarian tumours which vary greatly in their growth patterns and degree of malignancy. Many ovarian tumours are not cancerous and require only simple removal—fortunately these are the most common kind occurring in younger women. Ovarian tumours which are classified as cancers occur usually in women over the age of fifty. The age group in which cancer of the ovaries is most frequently diagnosed is between sixty and seventy. Ovarian cancer is the seventh most common cancer occurring in women, and is a major cause of death in older women. There are several factors now known to be related to increased risk of ovarian cancer:

Family history

Some forms of ovarian cancer are known to run in families. Having a mother or sister who has had ovarian cancer increases a woman's risk for developing this cancer.

Length of reproductive life span

Women who have early puberty and/or late menopause (fifty-five years or older) are known to be at increased risk.

Racial background

Ovarian cancer is more common in women of Anglo-Saxon or Mediterranean descent.

Number of children

Ovarian cancer is more common in women who have been infertile, never had children or had few children. The more children a woman has, the lower her risk of ovarian cancer. Having at least one child decreases a woman's risk of ovarian cancer by forty per cent.

Surgical procedures

There is evidence that *tubal ligation* is associated with a substantially reduced risk of ovarian cancer. Hysterectomy may also lower the risk of this malignancy.

The oral contraceptive pill and ovarian cancer

There is now conclusive evidence that use of the oral contraceptive pill containing both oestrogen and progesterone reduces a woman's chance of developing ovarian cancer. The protective effect occurs not only during the years the oral contraceptive pill is taken but persists for at least five, and possibly ten, years after the pill is ceased. Some studies have shown that the risk of ovarian cancer in women who have used the oral contraceptive pill is reduced to half that of non-users.

Controversial risk factors

There has been much speculation recently regarding the use of fertility medications in early life increasing the risk of later ovarian cancer. Several doctors at The Jean Hailes Centre are involved in studies now under way to resolve this issue. Another proposed risk factor is cigarette smoking.

Identification of these factors which increase or decrease the likelihood of ovarian cancer has resulted in varying theories regarding the cause of ovarian cancer. Common to these theories is that changes occur with regular monthly ovulation which predispose to the development of ovarian cancer. The important changes may either involve the structure of the ovary itself and the events in the ovary leading to ovulation, or the increased hormone levels that occur during the regular ovulatory cycle. Simply, the more a woman ovulates, the greater her risk of ovarian cancer. This is consistent with a higher risk in women who have had an early menopause, late puberty and no children and a lower risk in women who use the oral contraceptive pill, which prevents ovulation, or who have had many pregnancies.

The diagnosis of ovarian cancer

There is no screening test for ovarian cancer equivalent to the Pap smear for cervical cancer. *It is important for all women to have a complete medical check up every two years, especially after the age of fifty.* This should include a full review of any past medical history and a careful vaginal examination, even in women who have had a hysterectomy. In doing a vaginal examination any enlargement of either the uterus or ovaries can be felt.

Many women who have had a hysterectomy miss out on having a regular vaginal examination, however this is the best screening method available to detect the development of an ovarian tumour.

Vaginal ultrasound examination can be used to measure the size of the ovaries accurately and has been used in the assessment of women at increased risk of ovarian cancer. The ovaries normally sit very close to the top of the vagina and can be seen clearly by this technique—a very thin probe (sometimes described as being like a small microphone) is gently inserted into the vagina and the ultrasound waves produce an image of the ovaries on a television-like screen. This method only successfully detects about half of the early ovarian cancers and many are therefore missed.

More recently it has been found that a hormone called 'inhibin' may help in the detection of early ovarian cancer. Inhibin is produced by the ovaries during the reproductive years but is undetectable in the blood of post-menopausal women. Various ovarian cancers produce inhibin and blood levels of inhibin are elevated in women with these cancers. The leading research on inhibin and ovarian cancer has been conducted at the Prince Henry's Institute of Medical Research in combination with the Department of Obstetrics and Gynaecology at the Monash Medical Centre in Melbourne. The Jean Hailes Centre in association with these institutions is evaluating the effectiveness of the combination of vaginal ultrasound scanning and blood tests for inhibin and other cancer markers (CA 125) in the early diagnosis of ovarian cancer, particularly in women at increased risk.

Breast Cancer

Most women in the western world fear breast cancer. It is the most common cancer in women and the one causing the greatest number of deaths in women. In Australia in the 1990s *one* woman in *fourteen* will develop breast cancer during her lifetime. The number of cases of breast cancer diagnosed each year is increasing worldwide but the reason for this is not known. The increase has been partly attributed to the establishment of widespread screening mammography programs and heightened public awareness, but this is certainly not the whole story.

Most patients who present with a diagnosis of breast cancer have no known risk factors. *The significance of risk factors* has been discussed earlier in relationship to osteoporosis. It is important to understand that risk factors are determined by large population studies. Risk factors are less powerful predictors of disease in individuals as each person's biological make-up is so varied and complex. Identification of a breast cancer risk factor in an individual woman should be used as a positive step in prevention. This means regular self breast examination and in many cases more frequent screening mammography. The aim is *not* to label some women as having a pre-cancerous condition and certainly not to frighten anyone. Many women having known risk factors for breast cancer never develop the condition. This should be borne in mind as you read on.

Studies of various populations suggest that genetics and lifestyle factors contribute to the likelihood of developing breast cancer. Breast cancer in Japan, for example, is eighty per cent less common than breast cancer in Northern America. Is this because Japanese women are genetically less likely to get breast cancer or because they have a greatly different lifestyle? We do not know.

Research in developed countries has enabled the identification of various factors associated with an increased or decreased risk of breast cancer. These factors are broken down into the known high risk factors which increase the likelihood of breast cancer, the known low risk factors associated with reduced risk, controversial risk factors and postulated ones. The tendency for women now to delay childbirth may be contributing to the increase in breast cancer rate. Also the fact that the average age of the female population is increasing and *breast cancer is predominantly a disease of older women.* The majority of cases of breast cancer are diagnosed in women over the age of sixty with the occurrence in women sixty to sixty-five years old being more than double that of women aged between forty and forty-five.

Factors associated with an increase in the risk of breast cancer

- *Family history* of breast cancer in first degree relative, that is mother or sister.
- *Previous breast cancer* in one breast.
- A very small percentage of people who have a benign breast biopsy have changes associated with an increased risk of developing breast cancer.
- *Old age.*
- Living in *Northern Europe, America, Australia or New Zealand.*
- Having had *no children, or being older than thirty years of age* at the time of the birth of the first child. This risk factor appears to be more significant in women who also have a family history of breast cancer.
- *Having a past history of cancer of the ovary, endometrium or colon.*
- *Obesity in post-menopausal women*

Less important risk factors include an early puberty or late menopause, and short menstrual cycles over many years. City dwellers also have a greater risk of developing breast cancer compared with the rural population.

Factors associated with reduction in the risk of breast cancer

- Removal of both ovaries before the natural menopause
- Giving birth to one's first child before the age of twenty years
- Late puberty or early menopause
- Having five or more children may be significant

Risk factors for breast cancer considered controversial

- *Breast-feeding:* There is inconsistent evidence to support the belief that breast-feeding protects against breast cancer. This may be because the total length of time Westernised women breast-feed is relatively brief and any protective effect may require several pregnancies each followed by breast-feeding for a prolonged period. A very recent study has shown that women who breast-feed for a total of more than twenty-four months are at a slightly reduced risk of breast cancer in the pre-menopause years, however this study was unable to show that breast-feeding protects against post-menopausal breast cancer.
- *High dietary fat:* Recent information indicates dietary fat in adult women plays little or no part in the development of breast cancer. However, the fat and calorie content of the diet during pre-adolescence and puberty may have long term effects on subsequent cancer risk. In regions in China, where children have a lower calorie intake, and different composition of their diet, the average age of onset of menstruation is seventeen or more years. In contrast, in Australia the average age when menstruation begins is less than thirteen years and appears to be still decreasing. Energy restriction in early life may be significant by delaying puberty and therefore reducing the number of years of exposure of the breasts to higher oestrogen levels. Also diet in early life may have a *direct* impact upon breast development during puberty.

- *Alcohol consumption:* There is increasing evidence that alcohol intake may be an important factor in the development of breast cancer. Even small amounts of alcohol may be significant. Having three to nine standard alcoholic drinks per week may have a small effect but women who consume an average of ten standard drinks per week have a sixty per cent increase in their risk of breast cancer. Alcohol consumption appears to increase the levels of oestrogen, specifically oestradiol and oestrone during the menstrual cycle. This information makes it difficult to advise women about a safe limit for alcohol consumption. Perhaps the effect of alcohol is yet another factor causing the differences in breast cancer rates between the developed and underdeveloped countries.
- *Oral contraceptive use:* Past use of the oral contraceptive pill does not increase the risk of breast cancer in older women. There does however appear to be a *very small* increase in the risk of breast cancer in pre-menopausal women who take the combined oral contraceptive pill for four or more years before their first pregnancy.
- *Hormone Replacement Therapy:* To be discussed separately

Postulated risk factors for breast cancer

- *Cigarette smoking:* No specific relationship between smoking and breast cancer has been demonstrated.
- *Permanent hair dyes:* There does not appear to be any association with breast cancer
- *Anti-oxidants—Vitamins A, E and C:* There is no evidence to support the belief that taking supplements of vitamins E and C protects against breast cancer. *Women deficient in vitamin A are at increased risk of breast cancer* and they alone will benefit from vitamin A supplements. Vitamin A supplements however provide no benefit in women who have an adequate dietary intake of this vitamin.

Screening and detection of breast cancer

The simplest screening test for any woman is regular *breast self examination (BSE).* By getting to know the usual texture of her own breast, a woman can more readily detect any change. Virtually every general practitioner's surgery has pamphlets on BSE and these are also available from the Anti-Cancer Council.

Mammography is a simple low radiation dose X-ray investigation used to either screen women for abnormalities or assess abnormalities already felt. Screening mammography is performed on asymptomatic women in whom no abnormality can be felt. Mammography does not detect approximately ten per cent of cancers. Around the age of forty, women should have a base line mammogram performed and regular two-yearly screening should be done for all women after the age of fifty. Some women with a family history of breast cancer or with other specific indications should consider annual screening; this is usually individually recommended by their doctor.

Mammography will detect very early cancers before they can be felt, but sometimes BSE results in detection of a lump that cannot be seen on a mammogram. *A combination of BSE and mammography is recommended.* When a mammogram is performed it is necessary for each breast, one at a time, to be flattened between two plastic plates. Most women (eighty-five per cent in one study) describe the procedure as either 'comfortable' or 'uncomfortable but tolerable'. Very few find it a distressing experience. Sometimes an *ultrasound* is performed on a changed area of the breast to provide further information. This is a simple procedure in which the ultrasound probe, an instrument about the size of a small TV remote control, is gently passed over the breast and a picture recorded.

It is common for a surgeon to assess a lump by a *needle aspiration.* This means a fine needle is inserted into the area felt to be different and cells sampled are then examined by a pathologist. Although this sounds rather unpleasant it is a very simple, quick procedure with minimal discomfort. Suspicious lumps require surgical removal. Specific management of breast cancer is beyond the scope of this chapter.

The breast and HRT

This is an unnecessarily controversial subject too often discussed from an emotional perspective. The impact of the use of HRT on breast cancer is relatively minor in comparison to the far more significant impact of Westernised lifestyle on the increased frequency of this disease. It is also difficult to separate the use of HRT from the many variables known to influence breast cancer. Women who take HRT are more likely to have:

- consulted a doctor about a benign breast problem in the past
- to have had no children or only one or two and, if the latter, to have had children after the age of thirty
- to consume alcohol

All these are known risk factors for breast cancer. Furthermore breast cancer is not only the most common cancer in women, but also occurs most frequently in women over fifty years of age. Therefore most women taking HRT are in the age group most likely to get breast cancer. If breast cancer occurs in a woman taking HRT it should not be assumed that HRT was the cause.

When reviewing what is known about HRT and breast cancer, various things need to be considered:

- The duration of HRT
- The dose and formulation of oestrogen
- Whether progesterone is or is not taken
- Whether having other known breast cancer risk factors, such as a family history of breast cancer, alters any risk associated with HRT

Nearly all the studies of oestrogen use and breast cancer involve women taking *oral* oestrogen, most of which has been *Premarin* (conjugated equine oestrogen).

There is little or no information available regarding the use of other oral oestrogens, oestrogen patches or oestrogen implants and the risk of breast cancer.

Many studies have been conducted to ascertain whether oestrogen replacement is associated with breast cancer.

There is no data to hand that conclusively and unbiasedly addresses the question of HRT and breast cancer.

This is a controversial area and the subject of ongoing debate. All the studies carried out to date are in some way flawed* and currently we just don't have the answers. A consensus view would be that the postmenopausal use of HRT may be associated with a small increase in the risk of developing breast cancer.

It has been suggested that the diagnosis of breast cancer is more likely in women taking oestrogen as they attend their doctor more frequently and are more likely to have mammography. However, this only accounts for some of the increase in breast cancer observed.

- Very long duration of oestrogen use *may be* associated with a small increase in the risk of breast cancer.
- Currently available data indicates that *Progesterone taken for twelve to fourteen days each month is not protective against breast cancer. Progesterone taken alone does not increase the risk of breast cancer.*
- There is no solid data that addresses the issue of HRT use by *women with a family history of breast cancer.* Such women generally elect not to use HRT and therefore have for the most part been non-users in any of the populations studied. Therefore *no conclusions can be drawn regarding the use of oestrogen by women who have a known family history of breast cancer and its effects on their own risk of breast cancer. However, at this time it would be best to be cautious.* An individual's decision whether or not to use HRT will still depend on the severity of her symptoms and her personal needs and expectations and having a family history of breast cancer becomes yet another factor to consider in the overall equation.

Clearly further information is needed on long-term oestrogen use, the effect of different formulations, dosages and combinations of therapy and the relationship with female breast cancer.

Oestrogen after breast cancer

The use of HRT after breast cancer is becoming increasingly common. Clearly this is a controversial issue that must be discussed in depth by a woman with her treating doctors. Factors such as quality of life, whether or not the cancer has recurred after past treatment and the individual's overall prognosis need to be taken into account.

Alternatives to oestrogen in women with a history of breast cancer

- *Progesterone* alone can be used to reduce hot flushes and protect against bone loss. Provera, 10—100 mg daily or Primolut N, 1—10 mg daily are usually recommended.

- *Low dose* vaginal oestrogens can probably be safely recommended.
- Dietary calcium, exercise and other aspects of lifestyle should be reviewed as for any other woman.
- *Tamoxifen* is a synthetic medication used in the treatment of breast cancer. Although it acts as an anti-oestrogen toward the cancer cells and blocks breast cancer growth, it appears to have actions similar to oestrogen on the bones and cardiovascular system. Preliminary research shows tamoxifen reduces post- menopausal bone loss and cardiovascular disease.
- Low dose clonidine, a blood pressure lowering medication, has been used in the past to decrease hot flushes but the effect is in reality minimal or non-existent.

In summary, breast cancer is increasing in the world. There are probably many significant and interacting factors which need to be identified which are causing this increase. Exactly the part post-menopausal oestrogen use plays in the development of breast cancer does need to be further elucidated.

The fact that there is no significant increase in breast cancer incidence in women using oestrogen for less than ten years and in those who have used it in the past is extremely reassuring. It is also reassuring to note that no dose effect can be consistently demonstrated.

In the future, I believe lifestyle factors of women in the developed countries, particularly components of the diet, such as alcohol, will be found to have a far more significant role in the cause of breast cancer than currently appreciated.

---

*Most studies have been far too small to produce any conclusive data. Also such studies have involved women who have first chosen whether or not to take oestrogen and then entered the study. This means the women have self-selected their treatment resulting in 'selection bias'. The optimal study is one in which the volunteers are randomly assigned to be HRT users or non-users and then followed for several years. Studies conducted in this fashion have just recently commenced in the United States but their outcome will not be known for many years.

Chapter 6

NORMAL AND ABNORMAL VAGINAL BLEEDING

Normal Vaginal Bleeding

Normal vaginal bleeding, regular periods or menstruation are all terms used to describe bleeding from the lining of the uterus during the reproductive years. The special lining of the uterus is called the endometrium and hormones produced by the ovaries stimulate and maintain this lining tissue. During the normal monthly reproductive cycle, ovulation is followed by hormonal changes which prepare the lining of the uterus for pregnancy. If conception and subsequent pregnancy do not occur, the hormone levels fall and the lining is no longer maintained. It then fragments and is shed, to be renewed during the next cycle. This shedding process is the 'period' or the menstrual bleed. The average period occurs every twenty-eight days but commonly varies from about twenty-three to thirty-five days. Bleeding usually lasts about four days but it is normal for it to be as short as two and as long as seven days. Although most women feel they lose a fair bit of blood each month, the average total loss is only approximately 40 mls, or one egg cup full.

The menopausal transition

Leading up to the menopause, women commonly experience a change in their menstrual pattern. Cycles may vary in length, being either shorter or longer. Usually the first part of the cycle leading up to ovulation shortens and women frequently complain that their periods are occurring closer together. Menopause literally means the *last* menstrual period. For some women this means that their periods suddenly stop, without earlier warning changes in their menstrual pattern. Commonly, however, periods either become irregular or even stop for several months and for no clear reason begin again with apparently regular cycles. It is unclear exactly why this occurs, but women who experience this often describe classic menopausal symptoms such as hot flushes whilst their periods have stopped, followed by complete resolution of their symptoms when their periods return. While many women find that their menstrual loss becomes progressively less, others may have extremely heavy bleeding in the months or years preceding their menopause. Every woman has a different pattern because hormonal changes around the time of menopause vary from woman to woman and so does the response of the lining of the uterus in each woman.

Many of the menstrual cycles just before menopause are infertile cycles in which no egg is produced. However ovulation can occur unexpectedly and contraception needs to be continued throughout this time.

When is vaginal bleeding abnormal?

Women are all aware of their usual menstrual pattern, and equally aware of any change. Sudden heavy bleeding, often described as 'flooding' or the passing of blood clots requires medical attention. Heavy bleeding is commonly associated with increased menstrual pain, but absence of pain does not mean there is no underlying problem. Persistently heavy menstrual loss over several months may result in anaemia and iron deficiency and the earliest symptom of this is increased fatigue. Many women with iron deficiency experience weakness and lethargy before they actually become anaemic. A less common but curious symptom of iron deficiency is the craving to gnaw on solid things. People with iron deficiency have been known to crave for ice and to eat strange things such as chalk or even clay. This symptom of iron deficiency is known as 'pica'. These peculiar cravings disappear when the iron deficiency is treated. Treatment is two-fold—iron supplementation so that the body can replace the lost blood cells and diagnosing and treating the cause of the excessive blood loss.

Post-menopausal bleeding includes any vaginal bleeding that occurs twelve months or more after the menopause in a woman not on cyclical hormone replacement therapy. Such bleeding may indicate an abnormality in the uterus, although the bleeding may also be the menstrual loss following an unexpected delayed ovulation. Even if it is very, very light, medical assessment is essential to exclude cancer of the cervix or endometrium.

Common causes of abnormal vaginal bleeding

Pregnancy must always be considered, as unexpected bleeding may be due to a threatened miscarriage or an abnormal pregnancy such as an ectopic pregnancy. An ectopic pregnancy means that the fertilised egg implants and continues to grow outside the uterus. In ninety per cent of ectopic pregnancies the fertilised egg lodges in one of the fallopian tubes and continues to develop there. This is often described as a tubal pregnancy. The first symptoms of an abnormal pregnancy are usually abdominal pain or abnormal vaginal bleeding.

Uterine fibroids are benign growths or tumours that arise from the muscle layers of the uterus. Their true name is *leiomyoma,* they are the most common tumours in women and affect about twenty per cent of women over the age of thirty-five. Fibroids may occur singly but are more likely to be multiple and it is not known why they occur. Fibroids generally decrease in size after the menopause in women not taking oestrogen as oestrogen is known to stimulate their growth.

The majority of fibroids are asymptomatic, and detected only by routine vaginal examination, when the uterus is noted to be bulky. When a fibroid lies totally within the wall of the uterus, the main symp-

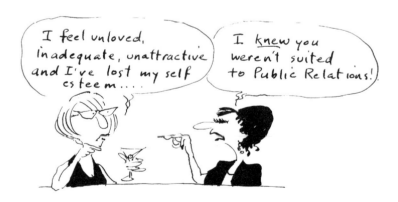

tom is increased menstrual pain. Some fibroids lie just beneath the lining tissue (endometrium) and cause increased and irregular bleeding by interrupting the lining and its blood supply. Large fibroids can press on the bladder and cause urinary symptoms.

When fibroids are suspected an ultrasound is usually the first test performed. This is a very simple test in which the ultrasound probe (like a small microphone) is placed on the lower abdomen and moved around to produce a picture of the uterus on a television screen. This is completely painless. Using the image of the uterus produced on the screen the size of the uterus and ovaries can be measured. The lining of the uterus can be seen too and its thickness measured. Any fibroids present are also seen and their measurements calculated.

In most instances fibroids do not require treatment, but when associated with either heavy bleeding or heightened menstrual pain, surgery may be necessary. Various surgical alternatives exist but the usual operation is hysterectomy, which means removal of the uterus.

Adenomyosis. This means that some of the lining tissue has migrated deeper into the muscle wall instead of remaining only on the very inner surface of the uterus. With each menstrual bleed the lining tissue trapped in the muscle layers of the uterus also bleeds resulting in free blood in the muscle which is an intense irritant and extremely painful. Typically adenomyosis develops in women in their late thirties, who have had children, and who develop painful, heavy menstruation for the first time. The diagnosis can now be made by sampling the uterine tissue (biopsy) using ultrasound equipment as a guide.

Cancer of the endometrium

This is the sixth most common cancer in women, and the twelfth most common cause of cancer deaths in women. The current lifetime risk of developing endometrial cancer is one in eighty-three for Australian women. This malignancy develops from the lining of the uterus and typically occurs in post-menopausal women, although it can occur before the menopause. The earliest warning symptom is abnormal vaginal bleeding. In women using hormone replacement therapy, erratic or unexpectedly heavy bleeding may be the first warning symptom, and indicates medical assessment is necessary.

Women who have continually high levels of oestrogen with low progesterone levels are at greatest risk of developing this malignancy. The most common condition causing continuously high oestrogen levels is polycystic ovarian disease. *Polycystic ovarian disease* is usually diagnosed in young women who have irregular periods and who sometimes also have a tendency towards weight excess, unwanted hair growth and, commonly, infertility. Women with this condition are usually recommended to take regular courses of progesterone to balance their relatively excessive oestrogen levels. *Obesity* also predisposes to endometrial cancer. Fat tissue produces weak oestrogens and consequently fatter women tend to have higher levels of such oestrogens. After the menopause, the weak oestrogens may continue to stimulate the lining of the uterus and after many years this stimulation may lead to the development of abnormalities in the endometrium and cause abnormal vaginal bleeding. Sometimes the abnormality is endometrial cancer. Continuous post-menopausal oestrogen replacement therapy, without progesterone, considerably increases the risk of endometrial cancer. *For this reason it is essential for women with a uterus to take progesterone either continuously or cyclically with their oestrogen replacement therapy.* The progesterone protects the lining of the uterus from over-stimulation by oestrogen. Taking combined (oestrogen plus progesterone) hormone replacement therapy therefore prevents the development of cancer of the endometrium. When *progesterone* is taken for a few days each month (called cyclical therapy) it is recommended that it be taken for *at least twelve days* and sometimes for fourteen days each month. In the past, women have been advised that seven days of progesterone is adequate, but this is now believed to be too little to be completely protective. Rarely, when a woman is unable to tolerate any of the available forms of progesterone, oestrogen is taken alone, but under constant specialist supervision and with annual sampling of the endometrium (see below).

Investigation of vaginal bleeding

When unexpected or erratic bleeding occurs, before or after menopause, it is essential that samples of the lining of the uterus are examined to exclude cancer. The traditional procedure is a 'D and C', or *dilatation and curettage*. This means that under a general anaesthetic, the cervix is widened (dilated) and the lining of the uterus is scraped out (curetted).

The tissue is then examined under a microscope by a pathologist who is able to identify any abnormal cells present.

A new procedure called *hysteroscopy* is now available to investigate vaginal bleeding. This is gradually replacing the 'D and C' as it is performed using only local anaesthetic, as opposed to a general anaesthetic, and an overnight stay in hospital is not required. Hysteroscopy is performed by a gynaecologist using the hysteroscope, a fine metal instrument with a camera built into its tip. The patient having the hysteroscopy lies comfortably on an examination couch. The hysteroscope, which is like a very narrow periscope, is passed through the cervix into the uterus and the entire internal lining of the uterus can be inspected using a television screen. Any abnormal areas are identified and specifically sampled for further analysis under the microscope. The samples are taken using a very fine wire which slides down the inside of the hysteroscope. Being able to see all the inner lining of the uterus and take specific samples of abnormal areas means hysteroscopy is highly sensitive, and probably the optimal test for the diagnosis of the cause of abnormal vaginal bleeding.

An alternative but less specific method for sampling the endometrium is the 'Pipelle' endometrial sampling technique. This involves passing a plastic tube (or catheter) into the uterus through the cervix and taking a sample of the lining through this tube. The lining of the uterus is not seen using this method, meaning the sample taken is less precise. However this technique appears to be as effective as the traditional 'D and C' in terms of diagnosis. For a woman who has had a normal birth, a hysteroscope or endometrial sampling can usually be done without the need for a local anaesthetic.

Summary

Abnormal vaginal bleeding is common and has many causes. The most important thing is that any unexpected bleeding, no matter how little, should be discussed with a doctor and a cause identified. This usually requires some tests. Because it is necessary always to exclude endometrial or cervical cancer, the earlier the diagnosis of either of these conditions can be made, the better the outcome.

Chapter 7

HEALTH PLANNING FOR THE FUTURE

A woman's health and lifestyle should be her own responsibility. The aim of this chapter is to provide an *outline* of the things every woman can do for herself in order to optimise her health and well-being and her quality of life after the menopause. As the years after the menopause now account for one-third of a woman's life she should be concerned about being fit and healthy into old age in order to maximise enjoyment of those years.

The health and lifestyle of the younger years will impact heavily on a woman's well-being in later life. Clearly women in their pre-menopause years, that is during their thirties and forties and really even younger, should think about the long-term effects of their social habits such as smoking and alcohol consumption, and health issues like diet, exercise and regular examinations like Pap smear tests. Life-long, people need to consider the short- and long-term consequences of their behaviour and plan their future with a positive attitude. Life does not end at fifty—for many it can mean a new beginning.

Psychological well-being

Most women go through the menopause around the age of fifty, at a time when life can be complicated by changes in the home and work-place. It may be difficult having to adjust to the physical changes of the menopause while trying to deal with the everyday hassles and changes in the immediate environment. Yet through this period of rapid change each woman needs to preserve her own self-esteem and retain, or maybe even rediscover, her own identity.

For some, the menopause may be a time of sadness, because the potential for pregnancy has finished and youth has disappeared. Germaine Greer writes about the grief some women experience for the loss of their reproductive years, and this sadness is often greater in women who consider the menopause to be synonymous with loss of sexuality and femininity. It is good to look back and experience nostalgia—this is very natural and, thinking about her earlier life, it is quite normal for a woman to feel both happy and sad.

Unfortunately the negative social attitudes that our society in general has towards older women doesn't exactly enhance positive thinking or self-esteem. Our culture tends to denigrate the aged, with such attitudes traditionally reinforced in literature, but more recently through visual media such as television, where older women are frequently depicted in a negative manner through advertisements and situational comedies. Society generally perceives older women to be inept, asexual and rigid in their outlook. Women are encouraged from their early years to embark on a lifelong pursuit of strategies to avoid the physical changes associated with ageing: the wrinkles, facial hair, drooping breasts and loss of muscle tone that society as a whole considers unattractive. It is important to feel beautiful (and certainly wonderful to look beautiful!), but quality of life and self-esteem are far more important.

Our society has a great deal yet to learn from Asian cultures which have far more positive attitudes toward the menopause and ageing. In such cultures the menopause is considered a natural life event and dealt with as such. The elders in the community are highly regarded and treated as competent and dignified individuals.

In our society many women experience a sense of relief in reaching the menopause, retiring from work and having time to pursue new hobbies. There should be time for a woman to look forward to new interests and spend more time on herself. The realisation that there are so many opportunities for self-fulfilment can lead to some women achieving lifelong ambitions.

At this stage in her life a woman may need time to accept the new life phase and to think positively. Knowledge of the changes that occur at menopause may help the adjustment and information may be obtained from books, magazines, pamphlets, videos and from lectures and discussion groups. Knowing that other women have the same experiences is often very reassuring.

The continual support and understanding of the family and close friends are necessary to boost confidence and lessen self-doubt. The menopause transition is like puberty in reverse, so if the family remembers that the woman may be experiencing similar feelings to the teenager, they can be more accommodating as well as caring and loving. The nurturing of the family unit has as much impact on the woman going through menopause as it has on the growing child.

Sometimes family and marriage problems that have been present in earlier years come under greater scrutiny and appear to be made worse by the menopause. Where there are sexual difficulties in a marriage, physical changes and other factors may precipitate a marriage breakdown. Psychological distress, such as depression, and social changes, such as the family leaving home, can all affect a woman's outlook on life. Marriage and sexual counselling often help at this time allowing for better communication and understanding. Sometimes a woman's anxiety or depression is so profound that psychological or psychiatric treatment is necessary. Women in this situation tend to have a past history of similar problems, the menopausal years causing past problems to resurface.

Open discussion of the fears of ageing and death is a social taboo. But most people on reaching their middle years are confronted in some way by their fears, this can be by the death of friends, debility or death of parents or sudden personal ill health. There are fears of illness, dependence, immobility and senility. We all dread loneliness, and the loss of friends and it is necessary for us to come to terms with the inevitability of death. Supportive relationships in which such anxieties and fears can be openly discussed are paramount to everyone's psychological well-being.

Dealing with stress

Stress is detrimental, whether it be due to work, family pressures or financial worries. Sometimes the symptoms of stress are subtle and may include sleeplessness, fatigue, moodiness and reduced concentration. It is important to be realistic and acknowledge when the pressures of life are becoming excessive. It is equally important to do something positive to decrease or avoid the stressful things or to develop strategies in order to cope better with life's difficulties. Many people benefit greatly by learning various relaxation techniques and incorporating relaxation into their routine. Everyone has different coping abilities and often the ability to cope can be improved by identifying and understanding the problem causing the stress. It is usually helpful to speak with someone who is emotionally detached from the immediate source of stress. This may be done informally, but professional counselling or referral to a psychologist or psychiatrist may be required. The main thing is to realise when stress is a problem, identify the cause and do something positive about it.

Nutrition

Diet has many roles apart from the nutritional value. The foods we eat and, perhaps more importantly, the foods we avoid have a far-reaching impact on long-term health and well-being.

The optimal diet should be:

- *Low in fat*—fat should only account for twenty to thirty per cent of the total amount of energy eaten each day and measured in kilojoules. A diet high in fat leads to excessive weight, heart disease and is associated with bowel cancer. Saturated fats which in the Western diet mainly means animal fats, should be limited. There is now a variety of less fatty cuts of meat widely available so a low saturated fat diet doesn't mean no meat at all. Major sources of undesirable fats are fast foods which are either plate fried in fats (hamburgers), or deep fried (for example chips, chicken and dim sims).

    Some fats are less harmful, and possibly even beneficial. Olive oil is a mono-unsaturated fat and inclusion of olive oil in the diet (cooking, salad dressing) has been associated with improved cholesterol levels. Fish oils are associated with better levels of blood fats and eating three or more fish meals each week has been associated with a reduction in heart disease.

- *High in fibre*—people should include plenty of cereals, grains, rice, fruit and vegetables in their diet. A high fibre diet not only helps keep cholesterol levels down and protects against heart disease, but also helps prevent cancer of the colon. Excessive fibre may lead to decreased calcium absorption so, as in all things, aim for moderation. Many people experience increased flatulence when they increase the amount of fibre in their diet, but this is only usually a transient discomfort which resolves when the bowel adjusts to the dietary changes.

- *Rich in calcium*—The amount of calcium in the foods eaten each day should be reviewed to keep the body in good calcium balance. Women usually need more calcium after the menopause (see chapter 3) and should try to include dairy foods and other good sources of calcium in their diet.

- *Low in salt*—It is not necessary to avoid salt, however, excessive consumption of highly salted foods should be avoided. Again, fast foods are usually very high in salt, which is probably a major part of their taste attraction.

- *Limited in alcohol*—There is probably no safe recommended daily or weekly alcohol level for women. In men, moderate alcohol has been shown to be associated with improved cholesterol levels but the data is less extensive in women. Consistently drinking more than two standard drinks per day (250 ml beer, 120 ml wine, or 30 ml of spirits) is associated with a significant risk of liver disease in women. It is also recommended that everyone has at least one or two alcohol-free days each week. Alcohol consumption may also increase a woman's risk of breast cancer (see chapter 6), and is associated with an increase in the likelihood of developing osteoporosis.

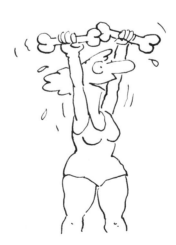

- *Adequate in iron*—Iron deficiency is probably the most common nutritional deficiency in our society. It most commonly becomes a concern during pregnancy, especially when a woman is in her third or fourth pregnancy. However, women who have heavy and/or prolonged menstrual bleeding are at risk of developing iron deficiency and subsequent anaemia, and should make certain they are eating sufficient meat or taking iron supplements to make up for their loss.

Ideally, everyone should not smoke and should avoid smoky environments. Smoking not only causes heart disease, lung cancer and emphysema, but it is also associated with osteoporosis and early menopause.

Controlling body weight

Women normally have more body fat than men. Unfortunately women of the 1990s neither like nor accept this. My impression is that most women's perception of their own body weight is usually five kilograms more than it really is, whereas most men think they are five kilograms less than their true weight! Aspiring to and achieving a body weight below what is considered normal for body height is probably undesirable from a health perspective. Very thin women do not necessarily have less heart disease, and are more likely to develop osteoporosis. *Women tend to gain weight at the time of the menopause whether or not they are taking hormone replacement therapy.* People generally lose muscle mass and gain fat with ageing. Maintaining a good exercise program (see below) will help keep weight under control and help maintain muscle strength.

Being overweight is undesirable. Obesity is associated with heart disease in particular, but also with breast and endometrial cancer. Controlled eating is fundamental to weight control. Sadly, Australian society appears to be becoming progressively more overweight and this trend is seen in children through to the elderly. In general, women should accept that they may gain some weight at the menopause but this should not be excessive, and if weight gain becomes a problem it should be dealt with.

A healthy diet contains meat (both white and red), fish, vegetables, dairy products, fibre, water and only small amounts of fat.

Exercise

Exercise is probably the most underestimated and least appreciated health practice available. For a woman in her middle or older years it may mean the difference between independence or immobility. Exercise is usually easy to do, it's getting her motivated to make the time on a regular basis that's the hard decision and then maintaining a program into her later years. It is a little like an insurance policy for old age, the premium being paid in hours of appropriate exercise.

The *benefits* of exercise include:

- *Improved well-being*—regular exercise enhances relaxation, increases most people's ability to deal with stress and has a positive effect on sleeping patterns.
- *Weight control*—a regular exercise routine plays a major role in long-term weight management. Contrary to popular belief, regular exercise usually results in diminished appetite, and the amount consumed tends to be more closely linked to the amount of energy being used. This is in contrast to sedentary individuals in whom eating patterns are most often dictated by social behaviour rather than energy needs.
- *Maintenance of bone strength*—regular weight-bearing exercise is known to help significantly in the prevention of bone loss and osteoporosis. Continuing exercise into old age will help reduce the risk of fractures.
- *Protection against heart disease*—regular exercise has been shown to improve cholesterol levels as well as lower blood pressure. These benefits, combined with any weight reduction achieved, can help considerably in the prevention of heart disease.
- *Stronger muscles and greater flexibility*—in old age a woman loses physical strength because the muscles become thinner, movements are more restricted, the body less flexible, and often the balance unsteady. All of these factors predispose to falling over more easily and fracturing bones such as the hip.
- *Lessening of menopausal symptoms*—A regular exercise program often improves self-esteem and may lessen anxiety and depression. Some women experience a reduction in hot flushes when they exercise regularly.

Walking, jogging, aerobics, golf and bowling are examples of the best kind of weight-bearing exercise. For maximum benefit, a woman should exercise three to four times per week for about forty minutes, the cheapest way being brisk walking. Swimming and other forms of non-weight-bearing exercise are good for fitness but will not have any positive effect on bone density or bone strength.

Medical check ups

Regular medical checks are recommended for every woman to assess her health to exclude heart disease, cervical and breast cancer as well as other diseases. A woman should see her local doctor every year for an overall review which should include a general health discussion and an examination including blood pressure, heart, breasts and an internal vaginal examination to check the ovaries and uterus. It is now recommended that a woman have a *Pap smear every two years* except when it is abnormal, then it should be investigated further or be repeated more frequently (see chapter 5 for details).

Mammograms or breast X-rays are recommended for all women, usually starting in the forties, but particularly for those over fifty. There are now breast screening programs for women fifty years and over, and the mammogram is performed every two years. Other screening tests which may be performed include blood cholesterol and triglyceride measurements and, when indicated, a bone density test.

Women should have a full knowledge of their past medical history, and if they can't remember it all, should write it down somewhere. Women in other countries commonly keep a folder of notes about their past illnesses and have copies of the result of any medical tests they have had done in the past. Women should understand why certain medical tests are performed and discuss the significance of the results of the tests with their doctor.

Prescribed therapies, whether medical or alternative 'natural' therapies should be discussed. *Women should be more enquiring and knowledgeable about their therapies.*

Every woman should:
- *know the names of the medicines she is taking and the dose* or have this written down somewhere
- *know why* she is taking the medicine(s)
- *ask about the known side-effects*

- *ask if there are any long term effects*
- *be aware that herbs, vitamins and mineral supplements are medicines,* and may have *side-effects and, if taken inappropriately, can be harmful.*

Life planning

The post-menopausal years are potentially the most positive and enjoyable time of a woman's life. It is important to start planning early, so as to maximise this life phase. A woman may think about her wishes, needs and ambitions and consider how they can be realised well before planning how to achieve her short- and long-term goals. Ideally goals should be set at different ages (that is a five or ten year plan) — normal practice in any well-run business! Perhaps the time has come for women to use business-like principles to organise this phase of their lives. For some women goals may include furthering their education, learning new sports such as golf or bowling, setting up a business, taking up new hobbies or travelling to new and exciting places. Other women may wish to extend existing activities. At fifty those women who are reaching their career peaks in business or in their profession, may wish to change direction or expand their present roles, whereas others may elect to spend more time with their family, particularly their grandchildren, or elderly parents. Maintaining communicating relations with one's family, partner and friends are very important for a woman's emotional, social and sexual needs and these don't disappear with age.

Lastly, financial planning for the post-menopausal years is a necessity. Seeking sound investment advice from a number of reputable financial advisers who specialise in people in their middle years is paramount, so that money worries will be minimised in old age. The post-menopausal years have the potential to be the most independent and satisfying of a woman's life particularly if she is physically and emotionally fit and healthy.

Chapter 8

MANAGEMENT OF THE MENOPAUSE—HORMONE REPLACEMENT THERAPY

When we talk about hormones we must first of all talk about glands. Glands are basically of two types—the lymph glands, present around the neck, in the armpits and in the groin, are part of the body's defence system and are what become sore and swollen when we suffer with a sore throat, an infected finger or an infected toe. These glands have no connection with hormones or the hormone system. The second group of glands are those which make chemicals which circulate in the blood stream and often produce very striking effects. Such glands include the pituitary, the thyroid, the adrenals and the ovaries. The hormones produced by these glands are necessary for our normal health and diseases result when too many or not enough hormones are produced. For instance, overproduction of the thyroid hormones produces the condition associated with toxic goitre and one type of thyroid hormone deficiency gives rise to cretinism.

When Hormone Replacement Therapy is discussed so too is the production of hormones by the ovary. During a woman's reproductive life, the ovary produces two major hormones, the female sex hormone oestrogen, and the pregnancy hormone or progesterone. The production of these hormones is not steady and regular but varies from day to day, usually having a fairly regular monthly and cyclic pattern. The levels of oestrogen in the blood, reflecting production from the ovary, are elevated around the mid-cycle time when ovulation occurs and are also elevated somewhat in the second half of the cycle, until just before menstrual bleeding. Progesterone is produced at very low levels in the first half of the cycle but its concentrations increase after ovulation, the second half of the cycle being dominated by progesterone. Each of these hormones tends to produce characteristic changes in the body, often detected as symptoms by a normal fertile woman. So the rising levels of oestrogen around the time of ovulation are associated with an increase in mucus vaginal discharge. The increase in progesterone is often associated with 'premenstrual' symptoms, including breast tenderness, bloating and fluid retention, and sometimes irritability and depression.

A normal and natural part of the ageing process in women is a marked decline in the production of hormones from the ovary. Starting on average about four years before the actual final menstrual period, the levels of oestrogen and progesterone produced by the normal ovary begin to decline and by about two years after the last menstrual period very little progesterone is produced and the level of oestrogen is less than ten per cent of what it was during normal fertile life. The concept of 'Hormone Replacement Therapy' is therefore a concept of replacing the hormones normally produced by the ovary when the decline in their production has given rise to symptoms, or when it may give rise to later complications such as cardiovascular disease and osteoporosis, as dealt with in other sections of this book.

The question is frequently asked as to whether such Hormone Replacement Therapy should really be considered as 'unnatural'. Logically it is certainly not unnatural. When any other hormone-producing gland becomes deficient it is good medical practice to replace the deficient hormone. Diabetics lack insulin, but there is nothing unnatural about replacing the insulin to treat their symptoms. People whose thyroid function has decreased, or whose thyroid has had to be removed, and who develop symptoms of thyroid hormone deficiency rectify this by replacing thyroid hormone. It is equally logical to take replacement amounts of ovarian hormones for symptoms caused by loss of ovarian function.

Patterns of Hormone Replacement Therapy

When we discuss replacing the ovarian hormones, therapy is divided into short-term and long-term treatment. Short-term treatment refers to the treatment of the immediate menopause symptoms such as hot flushes, dry vagina, irritability, depression and mood swings. Such short-term replacement usually needs to be given for two to five years. Some women choose to continue HRT beyond five years as they experience recurrent symptoms when they stop therapy. Classically these include vaginal dryness, low libido and hot flushes, but also many women describe diminished 'well-being', and prefer to continue on HRT. There should be no controversy as to 'how long' HRT is taken—it is a personal decision made by each woman according to her symptoms and needs. Everyone's experiences are different.

In contrast, long-term Hormone Replacement Therapy is therapy which is given for at least five years, often ten to fifteen years and sometimes for life. It is usually considered for the prevention of the long-term effects of menopause, specifically cardiovascular disease and osteoporosis—in both instances Hormone Replacement Therapy can significantly reduce the risks of these conditions occurring—it certainly does not abolish them. The protective effects of oestrogen against cardiovascular disease and osteoporosis are maximal whilst oestrogen is actually being taken, although some residual protective effects will persist after HRT is stopped.

Types of Hormone Replacement Therapy

1 Therapy with tablets

The most widespread form of Hormone Replacement Therapy in Australia is with tablets of oestrogen and synthetic progesterone (progestin).

Oestrogen Replacement Therapy with tablets can consist of the so-called natural oestrogens or of synthetic oestrogens. Natural oestrogens are those which occur naturally in the body, even though they may not be derived from a human source and even though they may actually be manufactured artificially. Because oestrogens are of completely known chemical structure and type we can make them in the laboratory and still call them 'natural'. The term 'synthetic' is used for oestrogens which do not occur naturally but which are nevertheless substances with properties identical to those of naturally occurring oestrogen. Examples of natural oestrogens which are commercially available as tablets include, *Premarin* (a mixture of several different types of oestrogen), *Ogen* (a particular type of natural oestrogen), *Progynova* (another similar type) and *Trisequens* (a natural oestrogen with some of the monthly tablets combined with a progesterone). Natural progesterone itself is not currently readily available for administration in Australia and hence synthetic varieties of progesterone are usually used where indicated. The two most common varieties which are used in menopausal Hormone Replacement Therapy are *Provera* and *Norethisterone* (or Primolut N). Sometimes the progesterone-only minipill is used as a progestin for HRT.

Two other progestins which are less commonly prescribed include *Duphaston* and *Androcur* (cyproterone acetate). Sometimes women who experience unpleasant side-effects with the more common progestins find these alternatives more tolerable. *Androcur* is a progestin with anti-androgen properties and its main use is in the treatment of acne, excessive body hair (hirsutism) and hormone-dependent scalp hair loss in women.

For women who do not have a uterus, as a result of having had a hysterectomy, it is current conventional practice to give the oestrogen alone, whereas for women with a uterus, a progestin is given together with the oestrogen in order to prevent the development of cancer of the lining of the uterus.

Tablets are normally taken on a once-daily basis often being initially recommended to be taken at night before going to bed to minimise any side-effects such as nausea. Nausea can result due to absorption from the bowel but generally, if it does occur, it is short-lived. Most women take their tablets at a time when they find it easiest to remember to do so.

2 Patches

A recent development is the ability to administer oestrogen through the skin by means of the so-called transdermal patch. In this form of treatment the oestrogen, 'oestradiol' is exactly the same as the major oestrogen normally produced by the ovary. Giving oestrogen through the skin avoids the need for the oestrogen to be absorbed from the bowel and to pass into the liver first, before being distributed to the rest of the body. This does carry theoretical advantages, particularly for people with liver disease or for those who would have an undesirable reaction from the direct effect of oestrogen on the liver, but the advantages are probably more theoretical than practical in most instances. Patches containing synthetic progestins are being evaluated in a number of studies internationally but are not yet available in Australia. The patches, currently available, are normally changed precisely every three-and-a-half days.

3 Implants

Another form of administering oestradiol, similar to that described for the patch, is by means of pellets actually inserted under the skin and delivering a dose of oestrogen for six to twelve months, depending on the dose and on the individual patient. This involves a very minor surgical procedure which is performed in the doctor's surgery taking only a few minutes with a local anaesthetic. Women who choose to have testosterone implants usually have their oestrogen replacement as implants as well, simply for ease of combined administration.

4 Vaginal oestrogen

When symptoms are particularly confined to vaginal dryness or are predominantly urinary in nature, oestrogen may be given by the vaginal route either as a vaginal cream or as a very small vaginal tablet. Such therapy is effective, safe and can be continued indefinitely.

5 Androgen Replacement Therapy

Androgens are the male hormones which result in the physical masculine characteristics. Androgens are normally produced by the adrenal glands and ovaries in women and circulate in the blood in low levels. In women, the exact biological role of androgens is unclear, but these hormones are probably necessary for maintaining muscular strength and muscle mass, body hair growth and bone density. They may also play a part in sexual arousal. After the menopause many women complain of a major loss of libido, especially women who experience menopause at an early age or who have their ovaries surgically removed. Androgen replacement will improve libido (only if the decline is due to hormone deficiency) and in many instances increase general energy and well-being. Androgens can be given as injections or tablets but the optimal mode of replacement is by testosterone implants six- to twelve-monthly. The aim of therapy is to restore the circulating testosterone levels to within the normal range for women. Used appropriately, testosterone implants are extremely effective, safe, and do *not* result in masculinising side-effects.

The modes of oestrogen administration

In women who have had a hysterectomy (as indicated above), it is current practice to give oestrogen alone, either by daily continuous tablet or by patch, implant or vaginal cream or tablet. For women who still have a uterus, the most conventional way of giving hormone replacement is by daily oestrogen tablets, or by patch, or implant, in combination with the progestin, which is given for ten to fourteen days per month. The most practical way to take the hormones is to start on the first day of each calendar month so as to make remembering to take the tablets easy. This form is called continuous oestrogen with cyclic progestin. It is the most conventional way to give Hormone Replacement Therapy, both for women who have not yet experienced their actual last menstrual bleed and for those within two to five years of the menopause. An alternative and increasingly popular way of giving Hormone Replacement Therapy, particularly to women who are more than five years post-menopausal, is by the so-called combined continuous method in which both oestrogen and progestin are given on a daily basis. This method of administration is designed to minimise the probability that vaginal bleeding will occur. In the conventional method in which progestin is given cyclically, most women experience a menstrual bleed in the two to three days following taking the last progestin tablet. In the combined continuous mode, the ideal result is the lack of any menstrual bleeding. In fact up to forty to fifty per cent of women will experience some bleeding or spotting in the first four to five months of

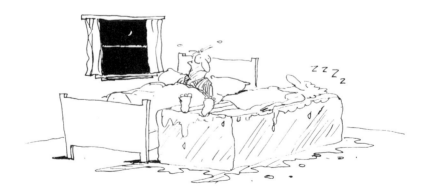

taking combined continuous therapy, but the majority will have no vaginal bleeding by the twelfth month and thereafter of taking such treatment.

The evaluation of the long-term safety and efficacy of combined continuous replacement has not yet been completed but as experience with this method increases, more and more women are taking their Hormone Replacement Therapy in this manner.

Side-effects

Oestrogens

Oestrogen therapy may be associated with a number of side-effects which are mainly of 'nuisance value'. They include nausea, breast tenderness, fluid retention and possibly weight gain. Side-effects are minimised by commencing therapy at an initially low dose and gradually building up to the full replacement dose, or by altering the timing or route of administration of the oestrogen. Women tend to gain weight around the time of menopause *whether or not they take HRT,* but naturally women blame HRT as the cause of their weight increase if they happen to be taking it. There is no evidence that HRT causes weight gain.

Progestins

Side-effects associated with progestins are the main problem associated with Hormone Replacement Therapy and generally mimic those associated with premenstrual syndrome as described above. Such side-effects include breast tenderness, bloating, irritability and depression. Again such side-effects can be minimised by giving the least necessary dose of progestin, by changing the type of progestin or the pattern or route of administration. In some instances, side-effects may be so severe that progestins are omitted altogether and oestrogen therapy is monitored by the regular taking of samples from the womb (see chapter 6).

Complications of therapy

The most controversial aspect of Hormone Replacement Therapy is whether it is associated with any increase in the risk of cancer. It has been well-documented that women who have an intact uterus and who take oestrogen therapy without any progestin are at increased risk of cancer of the lining of the womb, although the type of cancer tends not to be particularly malignant, and tends not to be associated with any increase in mortality. The taking of regular cyclic or continuous progestin completely neutralises the increased risk associated with oestrogen alone.

Of greatest controversy is the question of whether Hormone Replacement Therapy is associated with any increase in the risk of breast cancer. It must be remembered that breast cancer is a common malignancy in the Australian community with an individual woman's lifetime risk of developing the disease being approximately one in fourteen. A current opinion held by many experts is that therapy for up to five to ten years is not associated with any increase in risk, while therapy for more than ten to fifteen years may be associated with a small increase in the risk of developing the disease. However deaths from breast cancer are actually not increased, but decreased among women taking post-menopausal oestrogen. Assessment of risk versus benefit must be based on an individual's relative risk of fracture and/or heart disease on the one hand, and the possible small increase in breast cancer risk on the other. For those with either of the former risks, evidence strongly favours the advisability of long-term hormone replacement.

Indications for Hormone Replacement Therapy

Short-term Hormone Replacement Therapy is indicated when menopausal symptoms, such as hot flushes, vaginal dryness and psychological symptoms are troublesome, either during the time when menstrual cycles have become less regular or bleeding patterns have altered ('the menopausal transition') or in the first few years after the menopause. There is a very high probability that such symptoms will be relieved adequately with or without some side-effects.

Indications for long-term hormone replacement therapy include clear-cut evidence of risk of heart disease and/or osteoporosis with an increased probability of fracture. Identification of women in the second group, those at risk of osteoporosis, depends on bone density measurement. To assess whether or not a woman is at risk of heart disease, these are the high risk factors: being overweight, having high blood pressure, diabetes, a sedentary lifestyle, being a cigarette smoker, having raised cholesterol or low high-density lipoprotein cholesterol and having a family history of vascular disease (particularly premature death in a close relative from heart attack). These are the main risk factors for coronary artery disease, which should make an individual woman consider the likely benefits of long-term therapy. One particular reason to consider prolonged therapy would be if a woman had had a premature menopause, either spontaneously or as a result of having had to have her ovaries removed due to disease,

Contraindications to Hormone Replacement Therapy

There are probably no absolute contraindications to the taking of Hormone Replacement Therapy. The most frequent cause for concern is in the woman who has had a history of treated breast cancer and who presents with menopausal symptoms or increased risk of heart disease or osteoporosis. This area is one of continued controversy and a total spectrum of views can be obtained if authorities are consulted. There is, however, growing evidence that it is probably perfectly safe to use Hormone Replacement Therapy even after treatment for breast cancer, providing the controversial nature of the situation is clearly explained.

Active liver disease is certainly a contraindication to taking Hormone Replacement Therapy by mouth, though the use of the transdermal patch can be considered in this circumstance. A past history of blood clotting particularly when this has occurred spontaneously and in the absence of known risk factors is a cause for concern and needs investigation before Hormone Replacement Therapy can be considered. Again, in these circumstances, use of the patch or implants is generally regarded as preferable. Other rare medical conditions are occasionally listed as contraindications, though in many instances the data is not clear-cut.

Chapter 9

MANAGEMENT OF THE MENOPAUSE—'THE NATURAL THERAPIES'

There is no question that the use of traditional medicine has stood the test of time, whether it has been practiced in Asia, India, South America or in Australia. These days the practitioners are both indigenous people, whose use and knowledge of native plants and herbs is centuries old, and 'Natural Therapists' as they are known in industrialised nations. The power of these traditional medicines should not be underestimated and, as this is an area that has been researched very little, there is still a great deal we do not know about them. Alternative practitioners in Australia use a range of disciplines including:

- Nutritional advice
- Herbal medicine
- Homoeopathy
- Physical therapies such as massage and osteopathy
- Traditional Chinese medicine: including Acupuncture and Oriental Herbalism

The main alternative approach to menopausal management is the use of what are commonly known as the 'natural therapies'. This term can be misleading in its implication that other therapies including conventional medicine are unnatural, and this is certainly not the case.

Much of the advice given to a woman by her physician including modifying her diet, losing weight and exercising, could hardly be considered unnatural. In addition there is a multitude of modern medicines (something like twenty-five per cent) derived from plants and herbs.

'Natural' does not mean 'harmless'. Nature is not always kind. Any product which acts as a medicine may create side-effects. There is a small proportion of herbal remedies which can be toxic—particularly in untrained hands. They should be prescribed by someone with an extensive knowledge of their actions and side-effects but only in appropriate doses for specific individuals.

It is difficult to compare herbal remedies to conventional pharmaceutical products which have standardised purity and are given in exactly known quantities. Many herbs and plants contain multiple active chemicals with complex actions. The concern is often expressed that, because of this, herbal remedies are more difficult to regulate safely than a single purified chemical prescribed for its specific action. However, whole plant products often contain a unique balance of constituents which diminish the risk of side-effects or protect against toxicity. For example, willow bark (from which aspirin is derived) has similar anti-inflammatory and fever-reducing actions as aspirin, but because of the balance of its other constituents the whole plant does not cause stomach irritation or gastric bleeding.

It should be emphasised that these plants are being used as medicines, whether they be herbal teas or plant foods used as part of a therapeutic regimen. Like all therapeutic regimens, natural therapies must be treated with respect and supervised by someone who has expertise in the area as well as an overview of the patient's welfare.

Most practitioners use a combination of disciplines with nutrition, herbal medicine and homoeopathy being the main ones. Some practitioners specialise in just one area, for example herbalism, or homeopathy. What unites all the disciplines is a belief that the body has a great capacity for self-healing and the understanding that the medicines and methods used are supportive of the body's natural physiological processes. Supportive therapy is believed to enhance the body's own healing mechanisms and the return to good health. Practitioners aim to treat the whole person and long-term health is emphasised. Much of the advice given, including recommendations to avoid alcohol and smoking, differs little from the advice given by medical practitioners.

Natural therapies are not an alternative to the conventional treatment of diabetes, epilepsy, asthma, heart disease or major bacterial infections such as pneumonia or meningitis. Indeed, it is illegal for natural therapists to treat venereal disease, cancer, tuberculosis, diabetes and epilepsy.

Natural therapies can be used to improve the body's ability to cope better with a specific illness. By contrast, conventional medicine deals with particular pathology; for example antibiotics are used to treat pneumonia and surgery is performed in the case of appendicitis.

> The use of alternative therapies and conventional medicines is not mutually exclusive, but it is vital that every practitioner involved in the treatment of an individual knows what every other practitioner is doing and every medication the patient is taking.

Health Foods

Natural therapies should not be prescribed at the local health food store. Literally anyone can open up a health food shop, stock it with vitamins and minerals, herbal products (ranging from toothpaste and soaps to capsules and herbal teas), and give advice to consumers. In such circumstances the proprietor of a health food shop requires no training and there is no guarantee that the advice is valid or appropriate. You should not be consulting the sales person in the health food store about medicine for anything other than very minor self-limiting conditions.

The health food industry now has a $450 million per year turnover in Australia. It has become highly commercialised with marketing specifically directed at the health-conscious consumer. The health food industry is not answerable to an ethical body such as the Medical Board or one of the professional Natural Therapy Associations. The natural remedies available over the counter in health food shops and on supermarket shelves are regulated by the Therapeutics Goods Administration which has a special committee to deal with traditional therapies. Many of the available products, vitamins and minerals, not claimed to have specific medicinal effects are said to be listed and are labelled with 'Aust L'. Registered products carry the 'Aust R' label. Registration means that there is some evidence that the product so labelled has the effect that is claimed. Listed products are generally considered to be safe but require no evidence that they actually have the claimed therapeutic effect.

Management of the menopause with natural therapies

The alternative therapies differ in their methods but all treatment is considered to be supportive. A variety of foods, herbs, vitamins and minerals comprise the main medicines. Massage, acupuncture and homoeopathy are believed to stimulate the body's vital energies and muster a healing response. Treatment is very much of the individual.

It is often said that the natural therapists are not so much focused on the disease the patient has but rather on the patient who has the disease. The patient's constitution overall guides the choice of specific treatment, as much as their presenting symptoms.

In the management of the menopause there is no single formula for all menopausal symptoms. One woman's hot flushes may be treated with vitamin E, exercise and dietary changes whereas another may be recommended to take a combination of B vitamins and particular herbs. It all depends on what the practitioner perceives to be the basis of the individual's symptoms.

The following outline of strategies used to treat the menopause is by necessity generalised for the purposes of this book. Individualised therapy requires personal consultation with a therapist. Be suspicious of anyone recommending a single standard remedy for treatment of menopausal symptoms as this is not accepted as 'good' practice in naturopathy.

Historically the use of herbs and plants as medicines in traditional medicine systems is derived from practical experience. Over the last three to four decades there has been much scientific research related to nutrition and herbal medicines, validating many of these traditional beliefs. Clinical research is still incomplete, and practitioners use a combination of scientifically-based information and tradition.

Essentially there is little difference between the conventional medical and alternative approach to the menopause—both approach menopause as a transitional period. It is an adjustment period spanning some years, a time when a woman's body gets used to operating with lower levels of oestrogen and progesterone. Alternative practitioners use various treatments which support the body during these physiological changes and alleviate troublesome symptoms. Prevention of the long-term consequences of the menopause such as osteoporosis and cardiovascular disease requires long-term commitment by the patient and necessitates continual attention to diet, exercise and lifestyle.

Herbal medicines are widely available in a variety of forms and qualities, including teas, tinctures (alcohol extracts of herbs) and tablets.

Herbal teas available from the supermarket as tea-bags have probably little, if any, therapeutic value. Naturopaths usually recommend drinking specific herbal teas made from the loose leaves of the herbs. These are made rather like a China tea and their quality, unlike that of tea-bags, is such that a moderate intake of even three cups daily can have a therapeutic effect. Most European herbalists recommend liquid extracts of the plant called *tinctures* which are more concentrated and have a longer shelf life.

Tablets derived from specific herbs are also available. The purity of such tablets is fairly well controlled, however the quality and therefore potency of the original herbs from which different products are derived can be very variable. Often these tablets are formulated as combinations of two or more herbs and their effect may be modified by the interactions of the herbs used and depends on whether or not the formulation is appropriate for the patient's specific condition.

Herbal medicines may be used in a number of ways for treating menopausal symptoms. There are a large number of herbs which contain plant oestrogens which are called phyto oestrogens. These herbs can act like weak oestrogens within the body, occupying the oestradiol receptors. However, they are used in dosages which are much less than oestradiol which is produced by the ovaries and their metabolic activity is generally regarded as being ten to one hundred times less than most other pharmaceutical oestrogen compounds. Herbs containing phyto oestrogens include Squaw Vine, False Unicorn Root, Oatstraw, Black Cohosh, Red Clover and Alfalfa. Despite their relatively low content of phyto oestrogen and low biological activity they can be very effective in reducing menopausal symptoms.

Another group of herbs is believed to stimulate and support adrenal gland function and so enhance the body's production of oestrones. Among these herbs are Licorice, Scullcap and Dong Quai (Chinese Angelica) and Asiatic Ginseng (Panax Ginseng). *Licorice, Dong Quai and Asiatic Ginseng all require professional prescribing as they can be contraindicated in some women.* Excessive use of *licorice* can result in salt and fluid retention and elevated blood pressure. *Dong Quai* is contraindicated in women who have heavy menstrual bleeding or who take aspirin or anticoagulants. *Ginseng* is a very powerful herb which has been used for centuries by the Chinese. While the Chinese have great respect for its potency and use it cautiously, in contrast it is freely available and commonly used in Australia. When used either continuously and/or excessively, side-effects may occur and excessive use has been associated with the development of endometrial cancer. Ginseng should only be prescribed for a brief period and some patients are very sensitive to its effects. It should not be taken without supervision.

During the perimenopause, when the ovaries are still functional, certain herbs are believed to stimulate the ovaries directly. Such herbs include False Unicorn Root, Squaw Vine and True Unicorn Root.

In addition to these three main reasons for using herbal remedies herbs can be used as significant sources of minerals that are important after menopause. Herbal teas, such as Oatstraw, Chamomile, Valerian and Alfalfa, are said to improve the assimilation of and quantity of calcium and magnesium in the diet.

Nutrition

In general, natural therapists recommend a diet based on grains, fruits and vegetables, a diet which is low in fats, sugar and salt. They also encourage their patients to minimise the use of preservatives, additives and pesticides. Specific diets may be designed to either emphasise a particular food combination or to eliminate certain foods but fundamental to all the diets they recommend is the use of fresh produce rich in vitamins and minerals. When a natural therapist devises a diet the needs of the individual are assessed to ensure the woman has a diet appropriate for her individual metabolic needs and lifestyle. Specific strategies include:

- Encouraging foods rich in plant oestrogens, particularly soy products, linseeds and a variety of sprouts such as Alfalfa, Red Clover and Fenugreek. There is some evidence that a diet which has a high content of phyto oestrogens, adequate fibre and is low in fat can increase circulating oestrogen levels.

- Diet should be rich in calcium. Naturopaths also believe an appropriate calcium to magnesium ratio of 2:1 enhances calcium absorption (although the author has been unable to substantiate this traditional belief). For the calcium content of various foods, see Table 2 (chapter 3).
- Calcium absorption can be facilitated by a diet rich in saponins which improve the absorption of calcium across the gut membrane. Saponins are found in a wide range of foods such as legumes, soy products and herbs such as Red Clover and Horsetail.
- Substances which have a deleterious effect on calcium absorption and retention, such as caffeine, alcohol and nicotine, should be avoided.

The total dietary calcium intake, including calcium supplements, for a menopausal or post-menopausal woman should be at least 1200 mg a day.

In addition to the above, specific menopausal symptoms are sometimes treated with vitamins and essential fatty acids as well.

Vitamin E can be effective in the treatment of hot flushes and vaginal dryness. Long-term vitamin E supplements may also protect against cardiovascular disease. The recommended daily dose is 100—600 IU, starting with a dose of 50 IU and reaching the full dose *slowly* over a period of four weeks. Women with high blood pressure, diabetes or heart conditions are advised to take vitamin E under medical supervision, to use lower doses, not more than 200 IU a day, and have their blood pressure monitored.

Vitamin B6 (pyridoxine) can be very useful for the relief of fluid retention and sore and swollen breasts (mastalgia). It needs to be taken with a good source of vitamin B complex, particularly if taken long-term (more than four weeks). This facilitates its absorption and protects against the possibility of depletion of other B vitamins. The recommended dose is 50—250 mg per day. *Excessive consumption of vitamin B6 can cause nerve damage.*

Essential fatty acids: Evening Primrose Oil is the most well-known representative of this group of nutrients and is usually recommended for the treatment of breast pain, fluid retention, aching joints and premenstrual tension. Recommended dosage is 1000—2000 mg per day. It is expensive, however, and effective alternatives include *cold pressed linseed oil or safflower oil* 10—20 ml daily.

Safety of natural therapies

There is a false perception in the community that because these preparations are 'natural' they can have no adverse effects.

In general natural therapies are very safe. However *professional advice and guidance is essential if natural therapies are to be taken as treatments* and long-term. Inappropriate or excessive use of some herbal medicines and vitamins (as with conventional medications) can have *serious side-effects and significant health consequences.*

If it is not possible to consult a natural therapist because of the cost or because there isn't one available in the area, then consult your local GP. Many general medical practitioners these days are familiar with alternative therapies and certainly are able to assist with nutritional advice.

If you are taking a supplement or a herbal tea—or indeed any sort of vitamin or mineral supplement there are some important guidelines to follow:

- Make sure there are *no specific reasons why you should not be using this product.* Check labels for warnings. Talk with your naturopath or contact one of the professional natural therapy associations listed if you are concerned.
- You should expect to take the product for two to four weeks before you can find out for certain if it is helpful for your symptoms. Natural remedies usually improve symptoms slowly but surely.
- If you have any *ill effects* which you suspect are due to the natural remedies *stop taking them and consult a naturopath* or medical practitioner about their appropriateness.

If you are already taking medications—particularly for high blood pressure, a heart condition, epilepsy or diabetes, you should always seek the advice of a health practitioner before taking any other medications. Herbs, vitamins and mineral supplements are medications.

Finding a natural therapist

A reliable way to find a natural therapist is through one of their professional associations. This will ensure that the practitioner you consult has completed at least a three-year full-time course. This course includes studying the basic biological sciences. Relevant associations in Australia include The Australian Natural Therapists Association and The National Herbalists Association of Australia. Recommendations may also come from friends and from women's information services such as WIRE—Women's Information and Referral Exchange.

When a woman first contacts a natural therapist *she should ask about their training and experience in treatment of menopausal conditions.* She should also ask about the specific methods and therapies they use and how long each appointment will take.

Seeing a naturopath for management of menopausal symptoms is likely to be an ongoing commitment. The therapist may recommend monthly, or perhaps fortnightly consultations to begin with, for three to nine months, depending on the symptoms. As a patient, ask the therapist how long they expect the process to take as it is vital that you are comfortable about the course of treatment outlined and about your ongoing relationship with the therapist. It is also important to tell the therapist about any investigations already performed and the results of any tests done. Let your therapist know who your doctor is, and vice versa, as it is important that they can communicate with each other over the course of treatment they prescribe for you.

The medical profession is progressively becoming more aware and supportive of the alternative therapies, so don't be apprehensive about telling your doctor about the natural therapies you are using.

> It is to your advantage if everyone in your health care team knows exactly what you are taking.

Table 3 Foods/Plants rich in phyto oestrogens

- Soy Products—soy beans, soy flour, soy milk, tofu, tempe, soy sprouts
- Alfalfa sprouts/tea
- Linseeds/cold pressed linseed oil
- Fenugreek sprouts/tea
- Sunflower seeds

- Corn oil, Olive oil
- Lentils, split peas
- French beans
- Squaw Vine, False Unicorn Root, Oat Straw, Black Cohosh and Red Clover

YOUR QUESTIONS ANSWERED*

* Questions and answers were mainly compiled and written by Dr Robyn Craven on behalf of the Jean Hailes Foundation..

Q: Can hormone replacement therapy be taken as a short term measure or must it be taken for life?

A: Many women take hormone replacement therapy to alleviate their menopausal symptoms during the transitional years, without continuing on long term therapy. This usually involves 2-5 years of HRT.

Q: Can natural therapies reduce menopausal symptoms?

A: In many instances natural therapies relieve menopausal symptoms. Their effectiveness varies significantly between individuals. Natural therapies should be prescribed by someone with a sound background in this discipline.

Q: Can anything be done to ensure our daughters have healthy bones and are less likely to develop osteoporosis?

A: Young women need to have a sensible diet with adequate calcium, adequate but not excessive exercise and not smoke tobacco. Girls with delayed puberty or loss of their periods need to be assessed as such conditions indicate insufficient oestrogen which in turn may affect the bones.

Q: What about our sex lives after the menopause?

A: The majority of women do not experience any change in their sexual activity following menopause. Sexual satisfaction after menopause usually reflects how things were in premenopausal years. i.e. women who are happy with their sex life before menopause usually continue to be sexually satisfied. Some women experience reduced libido and vaginal dryness which can be treated.

Q: Does hormone replacement cause cancer?

A: Many studies have been done, particularly in relation to breast cancer, a common cancer in women. It is not known if there is a definite causal relationship between development of breast cancer and taking hormone replacement therapy but there may be a very small increase in the risk of developing breast cancer after 10–15 years of therapy.

Woman on hormone replacement therapy have less risk of cancer of the uterus than those not on hormone replacement therapy.

Q: Who should not take hormone replacement therapy?

A: Nearly all women are able to take hormone replacement therapy. However, certain conditions require specialist assessment before therapy can be considered safe. These include: cancer of the breast or uterus, a recent history of blood clots (thrombosis in veins or lung) severe liver disease or undiagnosed vaginal bleeding.

Q: What effect does hormone replacement therapy have on heart disease? Does it have any effect on smokers?

A: Oestrogen replacement therapy actually lowers blood cholesterol and makes it less likely for fats to be deposited in the arteries. Oestrogen reduces the likelihood of heart disease in post-menopausal women. All women who smoke should be strongly encouraged to stop.

Smoking has been shown to be associated with the earlier onset of the menopause and also is a risk factor in the development of both stroke and osteoporosis. Oestrogen may counteract some of the bad effects smoke has on the heart and arteries.

Q: How is hormone replacement therapy given?

A: Most commonly Australian doctors prescribe oestrogen tables to be taken daily. Preferably these are natural oestrogen such as Premarin, Progynova or Ogen. Non oral alternatives such as patches, implants and vaginal oestrogen are also available. The patch is applied to the skin of the lower body twice a week, whereas an implant (a small pellet) is inserted under the skin and lasts four to six months. In both cases the oestrogen is absorbed directly into the blood stream.

Q: What is the menopause and when can I expect it to occur?

A: The menopause is literally the very last menstruation of a woman's reproductive life. In practice the menopause is said to occur when a woman has not naturally menstruated for 12 consecutive months. Menstruation ceases because the ovaries no longer produce eggs and the monthly female reproductive cycles no longer occur. The average age for the menopause is 51 years with the normal range being from 45 to 57.

Q: How is menopause likely to affect me?

A: The most common symptoms of the menopause are hot flushes, night sweats, vaginal dryness, depression, anxiety, poor memory, poor concentration, insomnia fatigue, palpitations, decreased libido and muscle pains.

Q: Do all women experience symptoms at menopause?

A: No 10 to 20 per cent of women experience no adverse symptoms, 60 per cent experience mild to moderate symptoms and 10 to 20 per cent experience severe symptoms. In some women physical symptoms such as night sweats predominate, whereas other women may experience little or no physical symptoms but have significant psychological symptoms.

Q: My periods are regular still but I am feeling down and having problems with remembering things. Could I be menopausal?

A: Yes, that is possible as some women experience symptoms particularly psychological symptoms such as anxiety, depression and poor memory for several years before periods actually cease due to gradual changes in the ovaries with reducing oestrogen levels. This may occur over an average period of four years.

Q: I want my hormone levels done as I think I am menopausal.

A: Hormone levels are of relatively little value even if periods have stopped completely. This may be helpful to gauge the onset of the menopause when a woman has had a hysterectomy or if the menopause is suspected in women under the age of 40.

Q: I have had a hysterectomy but still have my ovaries. Am I likely to have an early menopause?

A: Between 10 and 20 per cent of women who have had a hysterectomy experience the menopause earlier than the normal age, on average about four years earlier.

Q: I am having problems with controlling my bladder. Could this be related to my periods stopping?

A: Symptoms such as difficulty with controlling urine and increased frequency of passing urine are generally considered to be part of the menopause syndrome.

Q: What are the best ways of coping with menopausal symptoms?

A: There are many ways of coping and it often depends on the diversity of the symptoms. Many women with mild symptoms cope with them without any medication or try natural therapies such as Evening Primrose Oil or vitamin supplements. Regular exercise is often helpful as it gives a feeling of wellbeing, enhances relaxation and sleep and may reduce menopausal symptoms. Women with more severe symptoms usually are greatly helped by taken hormone replacement therapy.

Q: What is hormone replacement therapy?

A: Oestrogen taken daily is the main hormone used to help menopausal symptoms. If a woman still has a uterus then progesterone given either cyclically, i.e. for 12 to 14 days each month or continually, i.e. every day is needed. Women who have had a hysterectomy do not need to take progesterone. Progesterone is needed to protect the uterus against over stimulation by oestrogen which could possibly result in uterine cancer.

Q: Are there other advantages from taking hormone replacement therapy?

A: Yes, oestrogen helps to protect the bones from osteoporosis and also helps to protect post-menopausal women from heart disease and strokes.

Q: What is osteoporosis?

A: Osteoporosis occurs when bones lose their strength and density and become fragile and fracture (break) more easily because of losing calcium. It is a disease that mostly affects women in their middle and later years. It is quite different to osteoarthritis which affects the joint surfaces.

Q: How does taking hormone therapy help prevent osteoporosis?

A: Hormone replacement therapy prevents the bone loss that occurs at the menopause. For the first 5 to 10 years after the menopause there is an increased loss of bone. Taking oestrogen stops this occurring.

Q: How can I assess my risk of developing osteoporosis?

A: There are several tests available for measuring bone density. The most common and safest are forearm bone density and x-ray bone density (DEXA). The DEXA method measures bone density at the sites of greatest concern–the hip and the spine—with very low dosage radiation. One in four women reaching the age of 65 years suffers a fracture due to osteoporosis.

Q: Should all women at the menopause have a bone density measurement?

A: No, each woman should be assessed by her doctor regarding her risk of developing osteoporosis and referred for a bone density measurement when appropriate.

Q: What are the risk factors for osteoporosis?

A: The most reliable risk factors are a family history of osteoporosis, early menopause, i.e. before the age of 40, a thin, small body build, being Caucasian or Asian, smoking and chronic alcohol and caffeine consumption, taking certain drugs such as cortisone for long periods, diseases such as over-active thyroid or anorexia nervosa.

Q: If I take calcium after the menopause will it stop osteoporosis?

A: No, although calcium is important after the menopause. An ideal daily intake is 1000–1500 mg, the equivalent of three glasses of milk. However, calcium alone will not replace lost bone. Oestrogen is the most important element in stopping further bone loss.

Q: Will taking oestrogen make me put on weight?

A: In general, women tend to gain weight around the time of the menopause whether taking oestrogen or not. On average, hormone replacement therapy users are thinner than non-users. It is important for all women to exercise regularly and eat a well balanced, healthy diet, including adequate quantities of calcium rich foods.

Q: What are the possible side effects of hormone replacement therapy?

A: The most common unwanted effects from oestrogen therapy are breast soreness and nausea. These symptoms generally improve with time or an alteration of dose or method of taking the treatment. Progesterone side effects include bloating, depression and mood swings, symptoms similar to the pre-menstrual syndrome.

Conclusion

Menopause is the natural conclusion to a woman's reproductive life span. It is an important transition time. Menopause is not something to be feared but to be understood.

Women who approach the menopause with positive expectations, good general physical health and equipped with some knowledge about the menopause can anticipate minimal disruption and change during this transition time and beyond.

Good health is fundamental to general well-being and should not be taken for granted. As well as becoming more discerning health consumers, women need to be more responsible for their own health. Good health requires long-term health planning and incorporation of preventative health practices into everyday life. The long-term consequences of choices made concerning diet, exercise, smoking and alcohol usage are ultimately each woman's personal responsbility.

Every woman has a right to make an informed decision as to how she wishes to deal with the menopause. Women should be supported and respected for their choices. Guilt should not be an issue.

There appear to be some misconceptions in which natural therapies are perceived as good, and conventional medicine and HRT as undesirable. There is no question that there are major physical, psychological and social benefits achieved when oestrogen replacement is used after menopause. Oestrogen replacement is no less natural than any alternative therapy, and should be considered an option for all women.

All women have the right to knowledge about their health, the right to make choices about their lifestyle and health practices and take responsibility for their life and health decisions, both short- and long-term. In order to do this women need to have self-esteem, and to look towards their future with a positive attitude.

Finally, a quote from Dr Jean Hailes' book, *The Middle Years:*

'At this stage of life, the middle years, both sexes have the world at their feet........Today, with the help of modern medical knowledge, they are able to feel well enough to make the most of life if they want to. I hope this book has been of some help'.